AF323976

AMBULANCES

A history of road, air, rail and sea ambulances
to the present day, with photographs,
specifications and diagrams.

64 Transport Series

AMBULANCES

by

L. GEARY

IAN HENRY PUBLICATIONS
1984

ISBN: 0 86025 879 3

Printed in Great Britain by
Whitstable Litho Ltd., Whitstable, Kent
for Ian Henry Publications, Ltd.,
38 Parkstone Avenue, Hornchurch, Essex RM11 3LW

CONTENTS

ACKNOWLEDGMENTS

The author wishes to thank the following for their considerable assistance in the writing of this book, particularly to Miss M N Slade of the British Red Cross Society; Miss Kate Arnold-Foster of the Order of St John; Mr R A Wilson of the Historic Aviation Service; and Dr Frank S Preston of British Airways Medical Services.
The British Red Cross Society; P & O Group Information; The Order of St John; Karrier Motors, Ltd.; Historic Aviation Service; Essex Ambulance Service; Talbot Motor Company; British Motor Industry Heritage Trust; London Ambulance Service; Bristow Helicopters, Ltd.; The National Motor Museum; The National Railway Museum; The Automobile Association; Loganair, Ltd.; V.A.G.(United Kingdom), Ltd.; Museum of British Road Transport; British Airways Medical Services; Hestair Dennis, Ltd.; Austin Rover Group, Ltd.; Southern General Hospital, Glasgow; B Walker & Son, Ltd.; Dormobile, Ltd.; Hawson Garner, Ltd.; Wadham Stringer (Coach-builders), Ltd.; Ford Motor Company, Ltd.; Vauxhall Motors, Ltd.; Mr B F Smith (The Daimler & Lancaster Owners' Club, Ltd.) for the photograph of the Daimler ambulance.

Military & Civil Ambulances

With the flashing blue lights and the intermittent shrill of its siren, the ambulance speeds along threading its way through the traffic, carefully, taking some risks, though not unneccesary ones, to its destination be it a home, a factory, a road accident, or returning to a hospital with the patients. Some seriously ill person needs hospital treatment, a casualty in an accident, a collapsed person in the street; what do we do? Simply pick up a telephone and dial 999 - Ambulance service, please - name and location of incident. The ambulance and its crew do the rest, the patient is in care and attention in no time at all.

Easy isn't it? Nowadays all taken for granted. We have just called an ambulance - but what is an ambulance?

The dictionary definition is "A special conveyance for the sick or injured; a unit of succour for wounded in the field; a movable field hospital." The definition does not indicate the type of conveyance, be it manual or mechanical, a man-handled carriage or wagon, horse-drawn vehicle or pulled by any other animal, a motor vehicle or even a stretcher carried by its bearers, could comply.

It is difficult to pinpoint the origin of this type of conveyance or even when one was first operated. In mediaeval times the dead, the sick or the injured could have been carried by sledge drawn by horses or men and this sledge may be termed 'an ambulance'.

When it was necessary to move the wounded from the battlefield, there was no service available to carry out this work. The wounded had to trudge or struggle along like an army in retreat. Some with leg wounds used sticks or even their own weapons upended with the butt under their armpits using it as a crutch. Sometimes one would fall by the wayside, to be helped up by his comrades, but if he could not rise and there was no room in any of the ammunition wagons or gun carriages, he was left to die - or occasionally a friend might shoot him to relieve him of his pain and misery, from which there was no hope of survival. Some were lucky and did find a place on a supply wagon returning to the base or a gun carriage on the retreat.

The ambulance, as a transport media, was developed for military use only, for the conveyance of the sick and the wounded from the battle front, around 1790 by two French army surgeons, Baron M Percy and Baron M Larrey during the Revolutionary Wars.

The early type was Larrey's 'ambulance volante', the flying ambulance, which in 1797 included the means of supplying the materials for the surgical treatment of the wounded with the advancing troops, as well as taking the wounded away from the battlefields after their wounds had been dressed. It was a two-wheeled cart capable of holding 2 stretcher cases. According to Baron Larrey's description at the time it was of simple construction and solid, yet light, and capable of rapid movement. It was drawn by two horses and considered suitable for operation in flat terrain. A second type was a four-wheeler, similar in construction to the other, but for mountainous areas. Both types had van type bodies with a rounded roof. Front and rear double doors were hinged at the sides, met at the middle when closed and fastened with a locking bar across both doors at the front and the rear. Two large apertures near the top of both sides of the body with sliding shutters inside regulated the ventilation. In the interior on the floor were two removable frames, on each a horsehair mattress and a leather covered pillow. These frames could be drawn out on castors fitted to each corner of the frames complete with mattress and pillow. The idea was to carry the wounded man upon the frame by means of iron handles attached thereon in a similar manner to a stretcher. The sides of the ambulance body were padded part way up from the floor and several pockets were provided for bottles and other needs. The second was similar, but

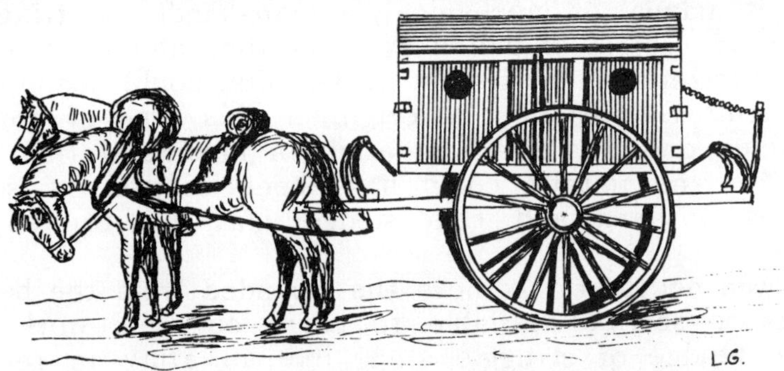

BARON LARREY'S "VOITURE d'AMBULANCE VOLANTE à DEUX ROUES" OR FLYING AMBULANCE.

had greater capacity. The ambulance body was slung by straps attached to the lower corners at floor level. The straps were each attached to one end of a quarter elliptic leaf spring, which in turn was fixed at the other end to the ambulance chassis. Each ambulance was drawn by two horses, one between the shafts of the

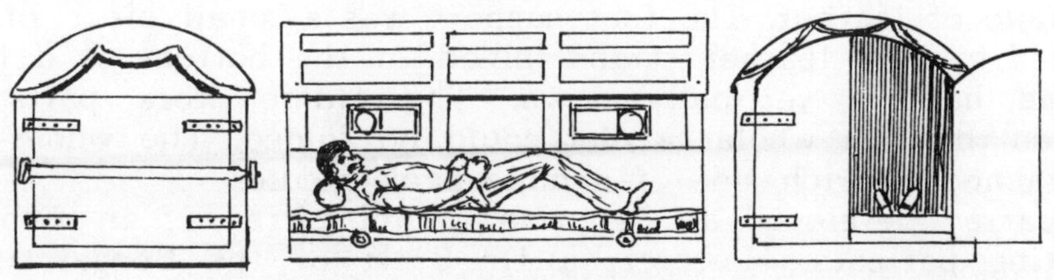

END VIEW - FRONT   INTERIOR   END VIEW - BACK
INTER OF BARON LARREY'S
"VOITURE d'AMBULANCE VOLANTE à DEUX ROUES"

vehicle and the other, on which the driver sat, was attached to a swingle tree.

One of the methods used by the French serving in Africa in the 1850s was the mule-cacolet and litière. These served in quite a number of campaigns and this method of conveying the sick and wounded to the medical base was very highly praised indeed. The use of mule-cacolets (mule-chairs) and litières (mule-litters) with the British Army was at the start of the Crimean War. The Principal Medical Officer of three divisions of the army at that time reported on the considerable merits of the French type cacolets and litières in their general application, especially on different types of terrain, where wheeled vehicles could not possibly function. Their construction was in the frame made from wrought-iron strips. A support for the back of the patient had a circular band attached to prevent the casualty from falling forward; straps and other parts

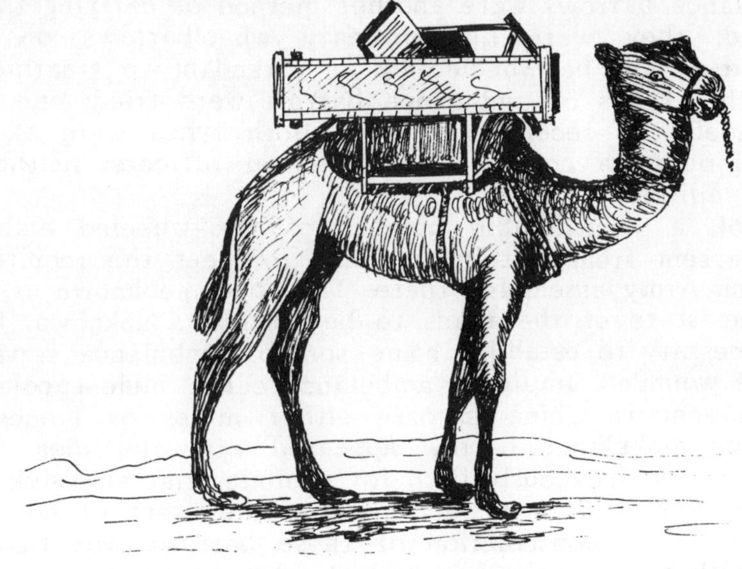

A CAMEL CACOLET FOR LYING DOWN CASUALTIES.

1839.

were made of leather. The foot support was a small piece of wood suspended by two leather straps joined to the bottom of a padded seat and hanging vertically down. The frame work parts were hinged so that the whole cacolet could be folded. The whole outfit was attached to each side of a mule pack-saddle.

Larrey developed an Egyptian Camel Litter as an ambulance for sitting patients. However, a Dr Brett of the Bengal Medical Service, Surgeon to the Governor General's bodyguard in 1839, built a contraption for the carriage of the wounded in a lying-down position for mounting on to a camel's back. The following is a description of its construction - "The main portion of the litter was a very light framework, adapted by its shape to the flanks of the animal; it was strengthened by iron bands. At the bottom of the framework and a part of the sides of the litter was filled in with canework, the remainder with strong varnished tent cloth. Inside was lined with cushions, a further light framework covered with doosootu cloth and painted white formed a shade or roof over the two litters, one either side of the camel. They were buckled to each side of the camel by means of thick straps made of buffalo hide. A strong rope passing through iron rings attached to the litter and crossing over the saddle further secured them to the camel."

Whilst Larrey designed and developed various ideas of types of ambulance to suit varying conditions, it was considered necessary to establish some sort of organisation to operate the ambulance. Baron Percy devised a military ambulance routine system, including personnel training in litter handling and stretcher bearing.

Ambulance barrows were another method of carrying the sick and wounded; they were like ordinary wheelbarrows on which soldiers could sit and be wheeled by an attendant to treatment. In 1856 two other types of ambulance barrow were tried; one having only one wheel, the second with two. Both types were examined and reported on by a committee of medical officers: neither was approved for military service.

In 1860 a considerable number of two-wheeled ambulance barrows were sent from Britain to China to meet the requirements of the British Army assembled there. They became known as 'China barrows'. The state of the roads to be used was unknown. It was, however, necessary to establish some sort of ambulance service for the sick and wounded. Improved ambulance carts, mule-cacolets and litters were sent to China in case either mules or horses were available. The ambulance barrow appeared with the idea that it might be used advantageously both for commissariat and sick transport with the aid of Chinese labourers, in the event of no animals being to hand. The construction of these barrows was that of a small cart with two wheels, two hinged sides, removable tail board, and open at the front; the shafts were such that it could be drawn either by a horse or a man. In this state it was used for the

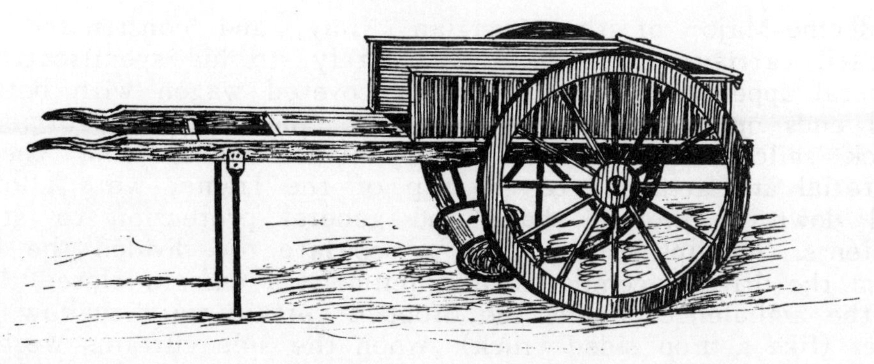

AMBULANCE BARROW (CHINA PATTERN).

carriage of supplies, but when needed for the transporting of casualties small adjustments were made – the tailboard was removed and the two sides were folded inwards on to the floor of the cart. The tailboard was laid across the front and secured. Two iron uprights, fixed to the rear of the cart chassis and having rubber type springs, were attached to the top of the uprights. One end of the stretcher was slung on the rubber springs and the other end put on two iron forks fitted into the shafts.

Jean Henry Dunant, a young Swiss businessman, was anxious to secure the interest and blessing of Napoleon III in a project in Algeria. There was a possible chance of gaining what Dunant wanted, but it was a question of how to approach the Emperor. In June, 1859, the war in Italy gave him the opportunity he sought, so he left his home in Geneva dressed in a tropical white suit and travelled to Apennine, a village of Pontremoli, from where a friend sent him to Castiglione, where Napoleon had his headquarters. It was here that Dunant saw, and was staggered at, the convoys of wounded being taken from the battlefields to undergo treatment. Dunant was further horrified to watch hundreds waiting, with no help, for the attention of doctors and surgeons.

Whilst through Dunant's efforts ambulances of a type – wagons drawn by horses that could take possibly two lying-down casualties – were instigated, his main concern was that an international force which, with the consent of every government, be formed to look after the casualties of war. He considered that, as a casualty, a soldier was no longer a fighting man and should be counted to be out of the conflict, to be protected by an International Force until either he was fit to return to duty or to be sent home as an invalid. With the results of Dunant's enormous efforts the Red Cross Society was formed. However, to look after the wounded some form of transport from a battlefield was needed.

In 1867 a horse-drawn ambulance was awarded the first prize for its category at the Paris Exhibition. Designed by Baron Mundy,

Médecine-Major of the Austrian Army, and constructed by M. Locati, carriage maker, of Turin, Italy, to his specifications. Its general appearance was that of a covered wagon with both sides and ends open leaving only a frame. The roof was formed from thick sailcloth canvas; the side blinds, made from the same material and attached to the top of the frame, were allowed to fall down to provide shade and general protection to stretcher patients. Curtains sliding along a separate rod divided the interior from the driver's compartment. Similarly, a curtain closed the rear of the ambulance. Below the dropped curtain were shallow wooden sides (like a drop sided truck). When the side curtains were rolled up and secured by tapes at roof level, the wooden sides were lowered. This gave access for the patients to be placed with the stretchers into the ambulance. The capacity was two stretcher cases and 3 or 4 sitting cases, or 8 to 10 sitting cases.

Around the 1850s a British ambulance to Regulation Pattern was introduced. The first of these ambulance wagons, as they were called, had unfavourable reports from the Crimea, so a committee was formed and met at the Royal Carriage Department, Woolwich. The committee inspected all the ambulances and conveyances submitted: steel springs and India-rubber springs were discussed and tried.

In 1866 the 'Fuller-suspension', the name for the India-rubber springs, proved defective in durability and was replaced by semi-elliptic leaf springs. The body of the ambulance was of the wagon type design, the cover being strong canvas on a framework of moveable hoops. In the upper part of the cover was a wicker basket slung from the framework to hold the men's knapsacks, and straps were attached to the sides of the wagon to carry firearms.

Although this wagon did well in its testing in England, it was not to prove successful when serving overseas.

It seems that the first time a horse-drawn ambulance wagon was used was during the Franco-Prussian War in 1870. Similar to the British wagon of the 1850s and 60s, it was fitted with semi-elliptic leaf springs and drawn by two horses. This ambulance wagon and others in the campaign were called 'English Ambulances' and bore a red cross on the sides of the canvas tilt: the fleet was operated by the Red Cross Society.

In 1889 the British Ambulance Wagon Mark V was introduced to the Medical Staff Corps. It was built to hold 12 men seated, or two stretcher and 4 sitting cases. Quite a smart wagon of the period, with a tilt cover offering good protection, mounted on a wooden frame. Similar ambulances were in service during the Boer War.

In the early days, the situation for the civilian population's sick and injured was very similar to those of the military. Generally, the doctor would be called to attend a patient in his home and, perhaps after examination, recommend that he be admitted to the infirmary or the workhouse hospital. The need to carry patients to hospitals was taken very lightly. Was there really a positive need to provide such a transport system at public expense? Many looked upon the ambulance as a military need and thought that when the wars were over ambulances were not necessary. This was not as surprising as it might seem for, until the wars dictated that something had to be done to move mass casualties, the country had managed quite well with practically no public ambulance service for the civil population, although there were always some private conveyances for those who could afford to be transported to private hospitals.

However, the need to move patients with infectious diseases, such as fever and smallpox, quickly and efficiently from their homes to the hospital was vital and in the capital it brought about the foundation of a London ambulance service, which was carried out by the Metropolitan Asylums' Board. The vehicles used were quite unsuitable, as well as being sometimes parked amongst tradesmen's carts after dealing with infectious cases.

In 1879 the Asylums' Board was given legal powers to provide ambulances for those infectious disease patients; the first of these ambulances were horse-drawn and looked more like hearses - black enclosed boxes. They took two stretcher cases and had a seat for two attendants. As before, the conveyance of those sick and injured in the streets and public places and patients with non-infectious diseases was still to be provided.

The earliest attempt in London to help such casualties appears to have been the foundation in 1882 of the London Horse Ambulance Service, the President being the Duke of Cambridge - but as the ambulances wore out they were not replaced and the service came to an end.

The Order of St John gave first aid instruction and provided litters and stretchers in parts of London, obtaining the co-operation of the Volunteer Medical Staff Corps and the police.

Accidents and sudden illness happening on the streets were dealt with mainly by the police, using hand litters or commandeering passing vehicles for help. However, the police did not consider this was part of their duty, especially when it took time which they could have spent in dealing with offenders to the law. In 1889 a member of a London finance house started a service, at his own expense, of 62 wheeled litters operating from police stations. The service was further supplemented by the St John Ambulance Association whose 35 first aid stations in London each had a wheeled litter and stretcher. Outside London also this subject was receiving a great deal of thought and in 1892 the members of a local branch of the Brigade of St John made a stretcher from a strip of canvas or blanket with two wooden poles as bearers and with two

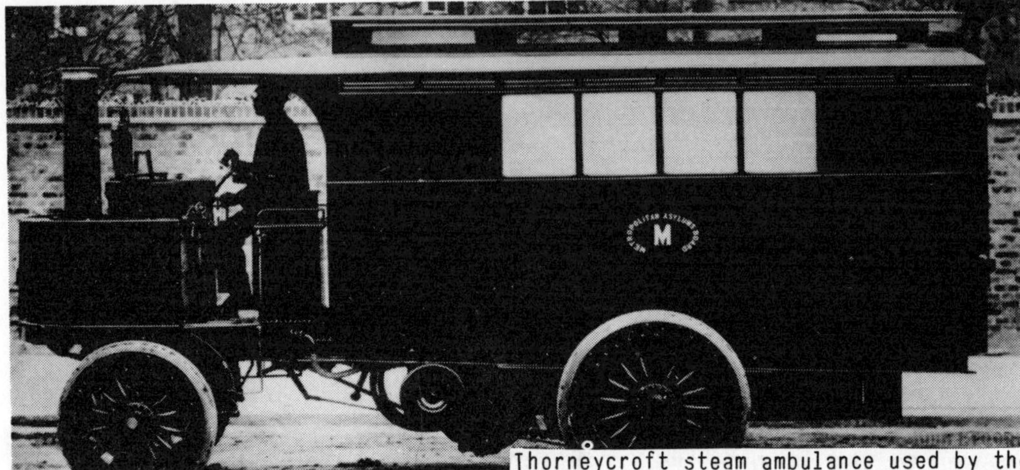

Thorneycroft steam ambulance used by the
(by permission of London Ambulance Service)   Metropolitan Asylums Board in 1903

spreaders one at each end. This stretcher they slung between two bicycles, which were presumably secured together by two spreaders across the cycles' crossbars. With the patient made as comfortable as possible and secured to the stretcher, two members of the Brigade mounted the bicycles and away they pedalled to the hospital. It worked – not elaborate – but an attempt had been made. In 1908 the first bicycle ambulance was produced by a firm in Morecambe, Lancashire.

An Invalid Transport Corps was formed at the end of the Nineteenth Century to convey the poor to and from hospitals and infirmaries, providing a service free of charge; infectious cases were not accepted. It is assumed that the better off patients were also catered for with either payment or donations.

John Furley of the St John Ambulance Association obtained a single horse carriage and converted it to be more suitable for the conveyance of the sick and injured. He had 4 attendants employed by the Association to assist in his transport operation. Furley went on to design better vehicles with improved features. He was knighted for his work in the foundation of the Ambulance section of the Order of St John.

When the first horse-drawn civilian ambulances were used difficulty was experienced with ventilation; the wagon was nicely covered with an elaborate canvas tilt and some other types, like converted vans, were all enclosed to protect the patient from the weather, but there was no ventilation or air circulation within the ambulance body and patients could become asphyxiated before they even reached their destination.

Modifications had to be made to ensure some comfort for the patients – softer carriage springs, rubber tyres on wheels and sufficient space to carry one stretcher or more, as well as first aid kits for on-the-spot attention and, of course, greatly improved ventilation.

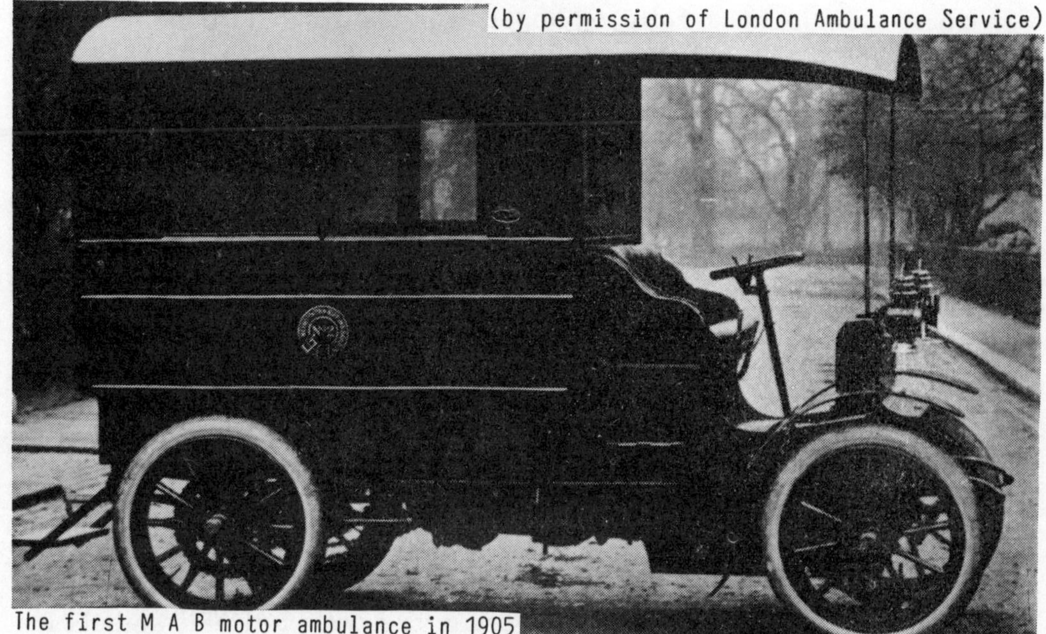

The first M A B motor ambulance in 1905

When the motor car came, it was a new era. Here was some-thing to help in the movement of the sick and injured and also to take the wounded from a battle zone quickly and with the chance of more comfort.

At the start of the Great War in 1914, the Order of St John and the British Red Cross Society joined forces and immediately set up an ambulance depot at Base Headquarters in Boulogne and were busy adapting the collection of motor cars that the public had placed at their disposal. In October, when the Joint War Committee took over from the Red Cross and St John, there were already some 120 ambulances, some lorries and a few touring cars in

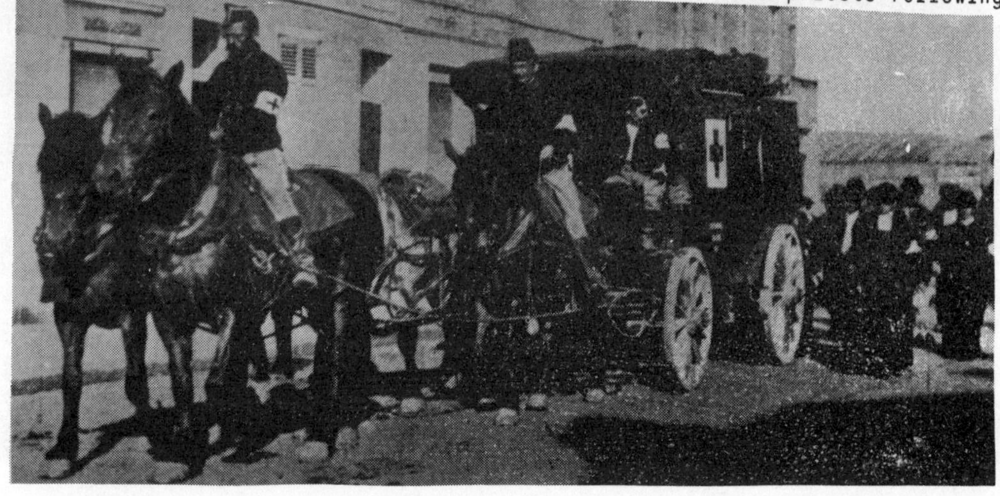
Red Cross in Flanders [bringing the wounded to hospital with priests following]

France. At Boulogne a fully equipped workshop had also been established to carry out repairs to ambulances and cars; the base was
often littered with broken rear axles, frames and springs, as well
as bodywork that suffered a lot of damage.

It was during this war, with its untold casualties, that it
became imperative to move the wounded from the vast stretch of
the front line to the base hospitals quicker than ever before.
Boulogne turned into one of the most important transport bases in
France.

The Royal Army Medical Corps were doing a great job, even
with their horse-drawn ambulance wagons. According to reports, the
hospitals in France towards the end of October, 1914, were
receiving something like 3,000 wounded a day.

The first motor ambulance convoy to be used as a unit was
sponsored by companies within the motor and allied industries. This
became a permanent unit within the Army Service Corps, under the
command of Captain Du Cros. There were 41 ambulances, 2 travelling workshops, 3 stores trucks, 3 officers' personnel cars and 10
motorcycles. The personnel comprised 5 officers and 144 non-
commissioned officers and men. During the war a field ambulance
was not just a vehicle for the transportation of wounded soldiers: it
was a large organised unit comprising a bearer division and a tent
division, altogether 234 officers and men and 66 horses. Its transport equipment included 10 ambulance wagons, each capable of four
stretcher cases or 12 sitting cases, or two stretcher and four

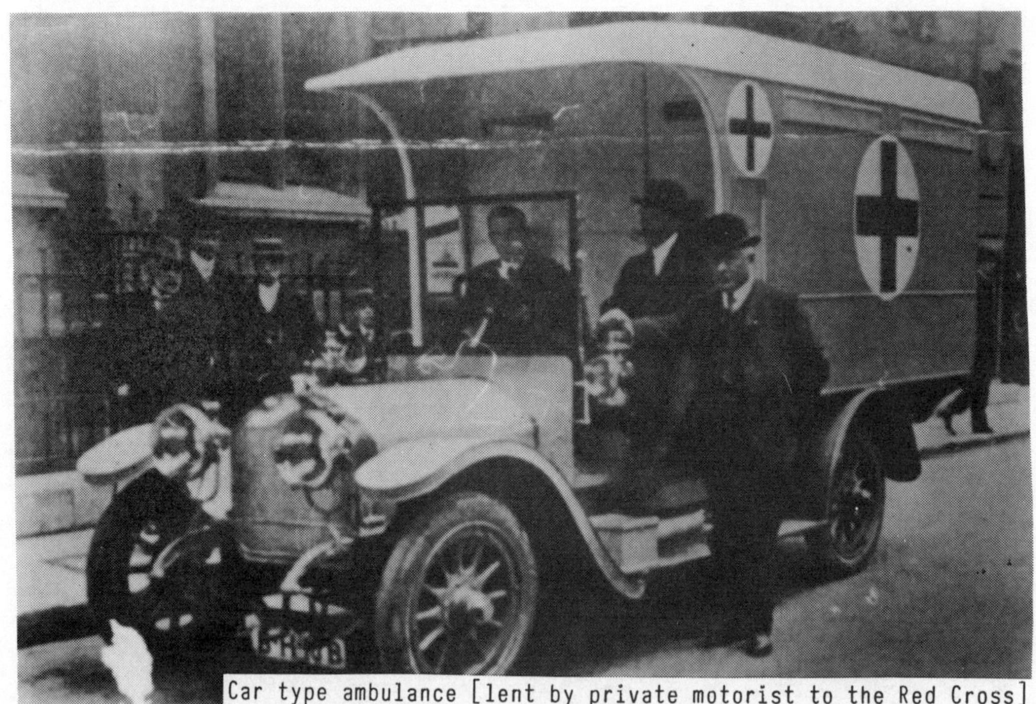

Car type ambulance [lent by private motorist to the Red Cross]

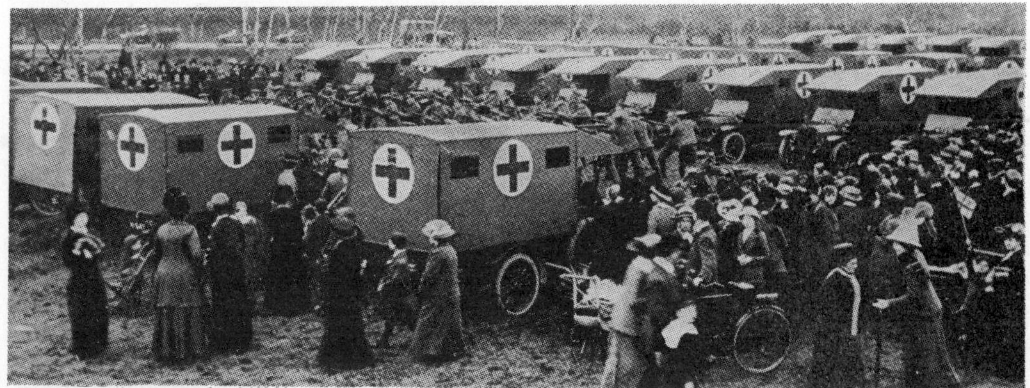

Motor ambulance convoy, 1916

sitting cases. The division was organised into three sections, each having six stretcher squads, with six bearers to each squad. It was the duty of the bearer division to collect the casualties from the field after a battle or, where practical, during the fighting to save time and lives. To each victim a specification tally was attached, giving name, regimental number and an indication of the nature of the wounds and the severity of them. In the ambulance wagons, the men were taken to the dressing station, which was formed by the tent division. This could be a series of tents or, if there was one available, a building.

The Red Cross did excellent work in providing motor ambulances and cars. They had 26, with a further 8 motor ambulances and 6 cars to travel the villages unoccupied by the enemy to search for the wounded.

Whilst such commercial vehicle manufacturers as Leyland, A E C, Dennis, Hallford, Commer, Albion, etc., already made vehicles for the fighting services, of which some were probably being fitted with some type of ambulance body, the availability of production for such medical purposes was limited. One of these vehicle manufacturers, Dennis Brothers of Guildford, made an ambulance chassis in 1915 – a 20/25 horse-powered specially built and also constructed an ambulance body. Two stretchers could be inserted, one either side, or one stretcher on the nearside with sitting patients on the offside; when necessary two further stretchers could be hung from the roof. However, something had to be done to keep the supply coming. Many of these vehicles received very rough treatment over unmade roads or streets torn up by shell fire. The demand came for more motor ambulances and the answer was mass production. Never before had casualties befallen any army in such a war as this: 40,000 men killed and more wounded in a single day was becoming a regular occurance.

In time the Ford Model 'T' (the affectionately-named 'Tin Lizzy') became the standby, in fact, it was at one time the only machine that could stand up to the cruel conditions imposed. At

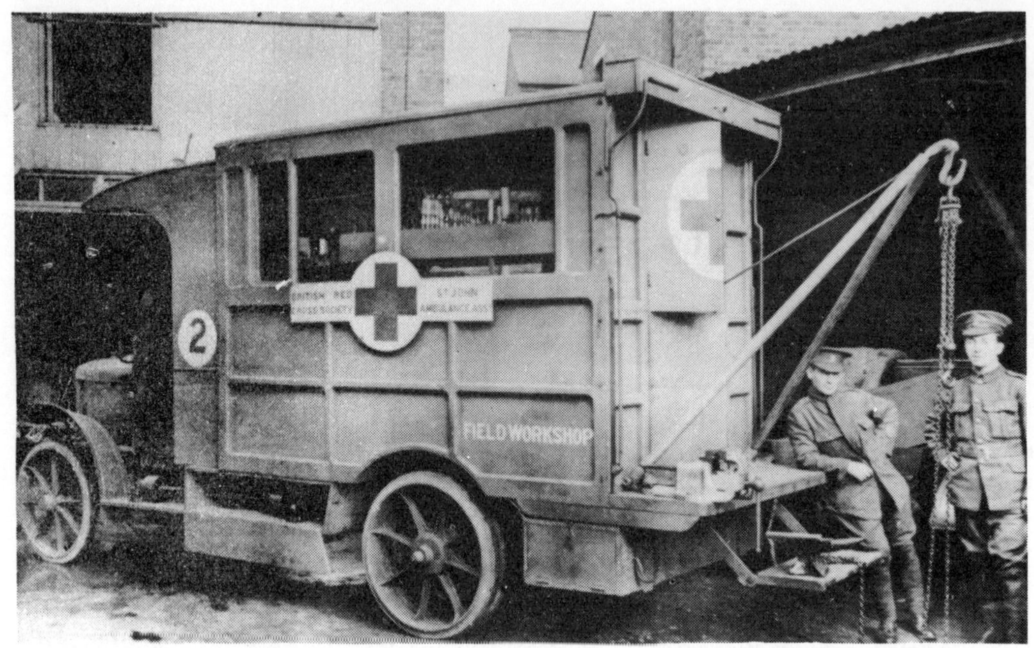

Commer mobile workshop, 1917

first the standard touring car went into action to evacuate the casualties; next, home-made ambulance bodies were built and fitted on to the Model 'T' chassis, front end version; later still, a specially built ambulance body, constructed from a wooden frame and canvas panelling was fitted at the Ford Manchester plant. Unfortunately, the body was not long enough to take the length of the standard army stretcher. The vehicle wheelbase could not be increased, because of axle loading problems, so 4 holes were drilled in the tailboard to allow the ends of the stretcher poles to protrude through, canvas bags being placed over the ends of the poles to stop draughts entering the interior of the body. This ambulance was capable of taking either two stretcher cases or four sitting cases, the maximum load being 344 kg (750 lb). These ambulances were built in their hundreds and did accomplish excellent work, being very much praised by both the medical staff of the base hospitals and the wounded soldiers themselves. Large cars, such as the Crossley 20/25 horse-power models, were used, again with an ambulance body fitted to the front end chassis version. This Crossley chassis was the same as that supplied at the Ministry's request to the Royal Flying Corps for similar duties and general service; it became known as the Crossley Tender.

Some very crudely constructed bodies appeared made from tongued and grooved wood boards, like a wooden hut, with two windows near the top of the sides. This type of body was fitted to the Commer 1914 truck chassis as well as the Ford Model 'T' and the Crossley.

In 1916 men were beginning to be withdrawn from such duties as ambulance drivers and orderlies to feed the demand for fighting men and their duties were being taken over by the women of the V.A.D.

Towards the end of the war some 3,446 vehicles had been sent to operate overseas of which 2,171 were ambulances.

After the war a Home Service Ambulance Committee was inaugurated and operated jointly by the Order of St John and the British Red Cross to investigate the civilian requirements of ambulances. Until then the concentration on medical transport had been for military purposes and no one had any real idea of the need for such a conveyance for civilian duties. In 1919 an investigation was made on the condition of the ambulances remaining in France and those which could be serviceable were brought back to this country. These were reconditioned by the Red Cross Society in their own workshop. County Ambulance Stations were organised where they were needed and where sufficient trained staff were available, it was to these stations that the Red Cross sent the reconditioned ambulances.

Improvements were made and in certain instances some attempt had been made to improve the travelling conditions for the patients; one scheme thought of was to suspend the stretchers by coil tension springs with one end attached to the stretcher rack and the other end to the stretcher poles. However, this and other attempts were abandoned as it was considered that the spring suspension of the stretchers caused them to move against the natural rhythm of the ambulance whilst in motion and such movements could be detrimental to the comfort of the patient being liable to cause a feeling similar to that of sea sickness and give patients a sense of insecurity. It was finally recommended that the stretchers should be rigidly attached to their racks.

When the British Red Cross Society and the St John Ambulance Association provided ambulance stations throughout the country, it was intended to be a trial service and not permanent, but it was only a few months after the experimental period when it showed that the ambulance service was proving a 'God send' to the invalid and for the doctors. Before a year had passed, the Society and the Association were convinced that, for the future, ambulance conveyance for the civil population must form part of their first aid service. This was the start of the National Ambulance Service in Britain.

Dennis Brothers became one of the most popular builders of ambulances, both chassis and body, with an intention to produce an ambulance that in every respect should be closer to the ideal than had hitherto been accomplished.

By 1920 a great number of ambulances had been distributed around for domestic service and it was considered necessary to issue a Register of Ambulance Stations, which was annually

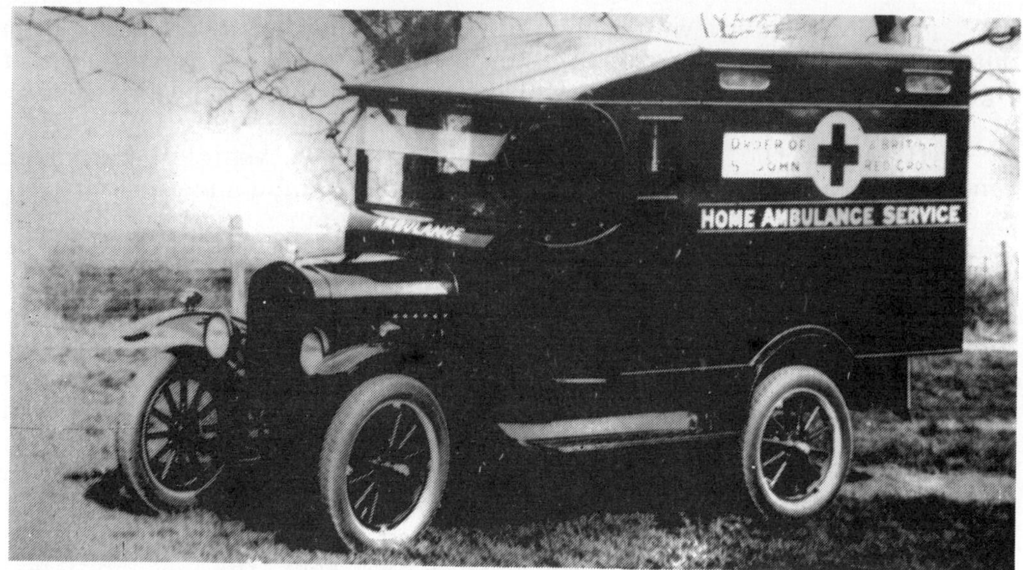

Ford Model 'T' ambulance, 1919

reviewed and re-issued for each county.

In 1920 ambulance bodies began to become more styled in their exterior design, but still without sufficient thought in the interior for the patients' comfort.

From the 1920s until 1939, whilst a number of ambulances were conversions of standard commercial medium range vans, manufacturers such as Vauxhall Motors (Bedford), Ford, Morris Commercial, Austin Motor Co. and Dennis Brothers built chassis cabs and chassis front end versions onto which ambulance bodies could be mounted. There was the Bedford 30cwt and 2ton normal control chassis front end and a comparable model of Morris

W & G Du Cros ambulance, 1926   (by permission of London Ambulance Service)

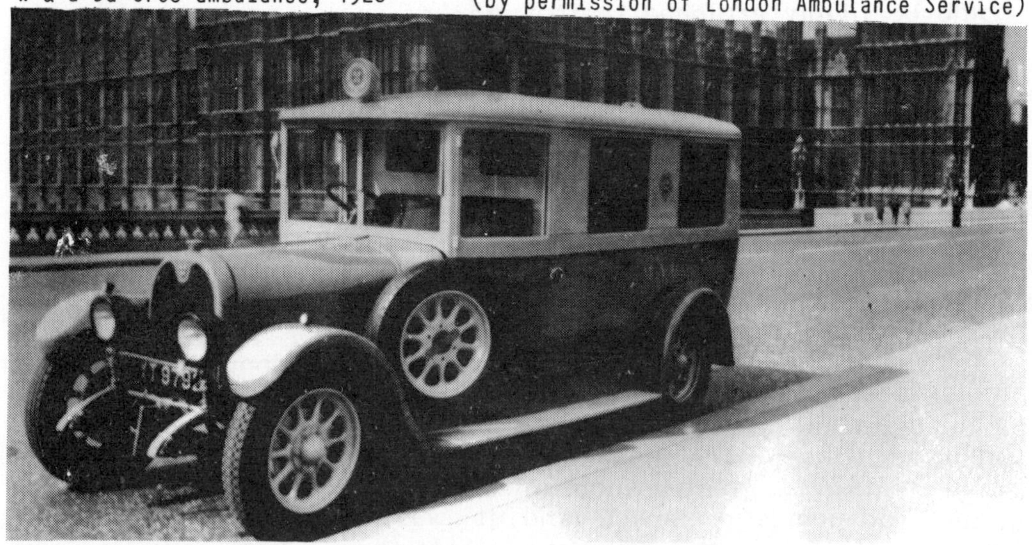

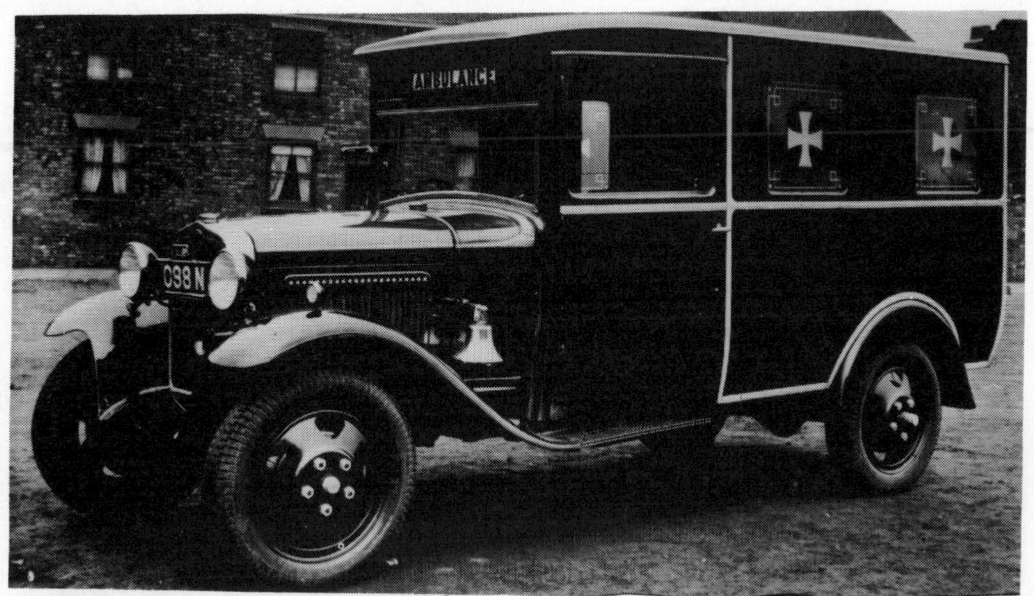

Ford Model 'AA' ambulance [St John Ambulance Association]

Commercial, both equipped with coachbuilt ambulance bodies. The Austin 12/4 chassis was another example on which a coachbuilt body was mounted. The Ford Models 'A' and 'B' chassis front end versions, as well as the 1930 Morris Commercial van chassis, making quite an attractive vehicle were all similarly equipped.

The Metropolitan Asylums' Board followed their acquisition of a Thorneycroft Steam Ambulance in 1902 with motorised units, such as W & G Du Cros. When, in April, 1930, the London County Council took over ambulance services there were 6 large ambulance stations, 107 vehicles and a staff of 270. As a result of this the General Section of the London Ambulance Service came into being separate from the Accident Section which was transferred from the Fire Brigade to the Public Health Department. Several more ambulances were acquired, one marque being the Talbot.

In 1932 Austin produced 12 purpose-built ambulances on their 12/4 car chassis, followed in 1935 by another three. Ford followed by the conversion of their Model 7V forward control 2ton van and a purpose-built body on the front end chassis version. Quite a number of Bedford and Morris Commercial ambulances were supplied to the British Red Cross.

In 1934 an ambulance body was mounted by Herbert Lomas coachbuilders on a Leyland 'Cub' chassis and it is believed that 6 were supplied to Liverpool.

In the early part of 1939 war was again imminent and by September St John Ambulance Association and the British Red Cross Society had made a formal agreement with the War Office to carry out joint services and set up the Transport of the Wounded Department for overseas service.

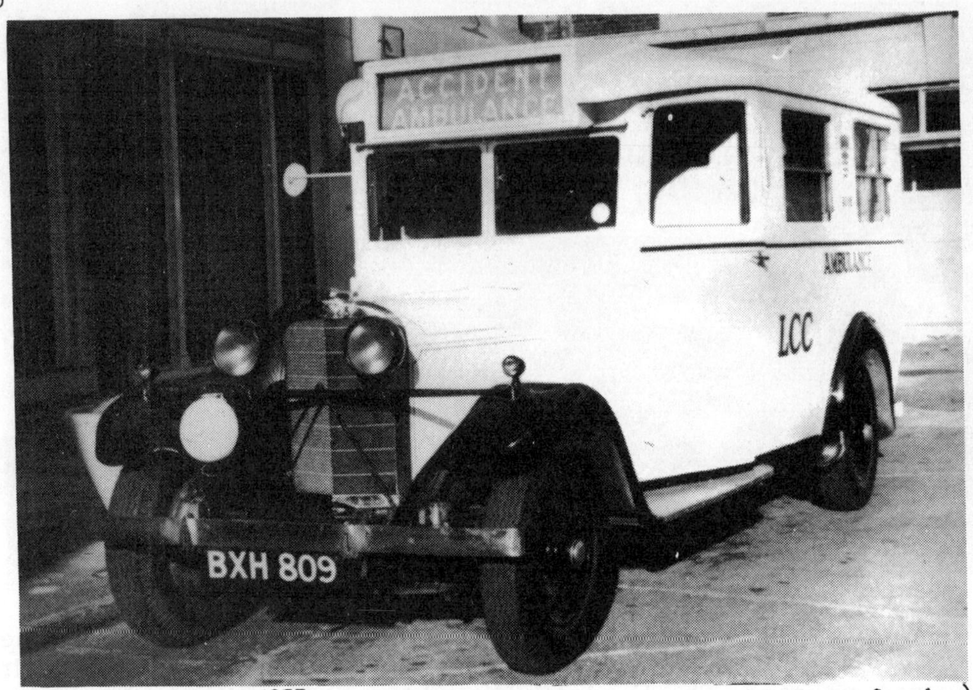

Talbot ambulance, 1935   (by permission of London Ambulance Service)

On 3 September war was declared and every available motor manufacturer turned over its production to either War Office transport and fighting vehicles or to tanks and munitions. Ford large 2 ton chassis front end version fitted with a 4 stretcher ambulance body, Model RO1T was produced, together with Bedford's 30cwt and 2ton chassis fitted with similar capacity ambulance bodies. These were followed by quite a number of Morris Commercial and Austin ambulances. Other manufacturers produced such vehicles where the capacity was available. The 15cwt military general service and infantry truck produced by Ford, Bedford, Morris Commercial and Humber were also used for other roles for the Home Front, including that of ambulances. There was also the Ford 10cwt van, the Model E83W, converted into a small ambulance as part of its many variations.

By March, 1940, there were enough ambulances and ancillary vehicles to form an ambulance unit to ship to the British Red Cross Commission in France. Unfortunately, all these vehicles were lost before and during the evacuation at Dunkirk.

In June, 1940, the War Organisation, realising the need for ambulances at home, especially for the conveyance of casualties as a result of anticipated enemy air raids and to back up the ambulance trains in the event of mass evacuation of any of the country's towns or cities, informed the military authorities that a number of motor ambulances and crews would have to be placed at the disposal for duties on the Home Front. Within 6 months 131 ambul-

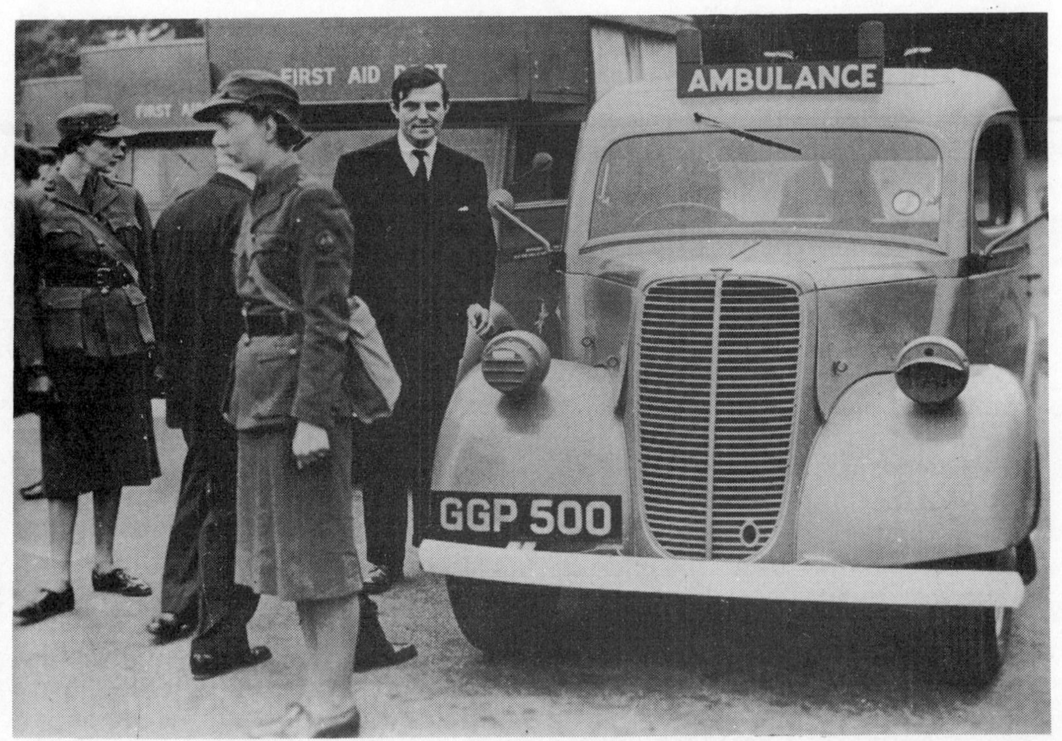

Ford Model E83W small ambulance, 1940

ances were operating within the Home Commands.

The War Organisation's Transport of Wounded Department had three main functions: that of supply, maintenance and equipment; personnel recruitment and training; and administration and the control of the Home Units working with the Service Authorities. Also there was the actual operation and staffing of certain other Home Ambulance Services, mobile X-ray units and physiotherapy vans, etc. St John Ambulance and Red Cross joint ambulance service, together with others under the Air Raid Precautions authorities, toiled day and night evacuating and attending to air raid victims throughout the country.

By 1945 ambulances and other ancillary vehicles distributed totalled some 2,000 home-based and 752 actively engaged overseas.Maintenance, fuel, and oil were provided by the army, including rations and accommodation for the personnel, together with the issue of steel helmets, respirators and capes. During the course of the war these ambulances and crews conveyed and gave attention to 681,530 casualties.

A number of ambulances and crews were stationed at Swindon to take care of the casualties arriving by air ambulance and other types of aircraft. Others were stationed with their crews at Hythe and Burgess Hill, near Brighton. The arrival of casualties at Swindon were very frequent, with no scheduled times they simply touched down one after another, working the air crews, nurses and ambulance drivers and attendants continually round the clock. To ensure that there were sufficient drivers to try to maintain the service, as well as offering some rest, drivers were recruited from voluntary organisations, including those available from Commonwealth volunteer units stationed in Britain and the Women's Transport Service of the First Aid Nursing Yeomanry. There is no doubt that these ambulances all over the country at receiving stations achieved a great performance including those carrying from coastal areas many injured, wounded, or exhausted, survivors from ships damaged or sunk by enemy action.

The degree of ambulance dependability demands a high standard from the drivers and the War Organisation demanded such standards. Training and testing were severe – as they should be, for lives depended on their skill.

After the Second World War transport of all kinds was under review and badly needed replacing, including ambulances for both military and civilian duties. A great number of ambulances had been lost during hostilities. Ambulances with a low mileage on the tachometer were transferred from the Home Commands in the country to the Home Ambulance Service Department: those overseas were inspected and, if in reasonable condition or repairable, were given to the Allied Red Cross Societies, who were in need of all kinds of transport. 350 ambulances in London alone were stripped to chassis, then serviced, repaired and painted. The old wood-framed bodies were scrapped and replaced by coachbuilt types equipped for peacetime activities. Those with mileages in excess of 50,000 miles and/or having defects were sold by public auction. The rehabilitation of these wartime ambulances was completed in 1948, the cost coming to £115,000.

In 1946 several motor ambulances were introduced built on standard commercial chassis, such as the Ford 7V, Bedford, Morris Commercial and Austin; in 1948 the Daimler Motor Company (now part of the Jaguar group) brought in a new high-class ambulance that continued in production until 1962. This Daimler ambulance was another attempt to produce the 'perfect' vehicle. A generous power to weight ratio, which meant a good vehicle performance, was provided by the Daimler 6 cylinder petrol engine developing 110 b.h.p at 3,600 r.p.m. and a carefully designed lightweight chassis. The pre-selector gearbox and fluid flywheel coupling made driving less tiring and with a smooth take-off. Acceleration was good, as was maximum speed, while climbability up reasonably steep gradients achieved excellent results. The ambulance body was designed and built by Barker & Co. (Coachbuilders), for Hooper & Co., who at the time owned the company: other high class body builders supplied ambulance bodies for the chassis. The construction of the chassis frame was box section, with cruciform type crossmembers,

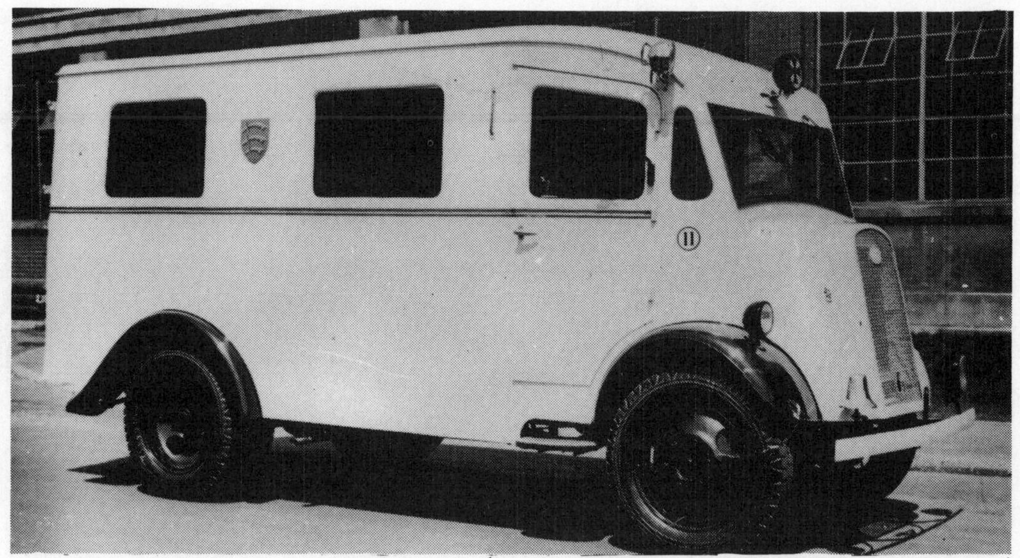

Ford Model 7V ambulance, 1946   (by permission of Essex Ambulance Service)

producing a strong and lightweight structure.

The effective fleet operated by the Red Cross and the St John Ambulance Voluntary Units was now over 1,000 in the British Isles; Bedford supplied quite a number of new machines to the British Red Cross in 1948.

In 1947 when India was split, actrocities were so bad that one country, Pakistan, accepted the Red Cross Society's offer of help with enthusiasm. The Medical Commission was sent out to establish hospitals in several towns, together with an ambulance brigade, including a mobile dispensary and other vehicles.

In 1948 the introduction of the National Health Service in Britain caused the responsibility for the provision of ambulances and other welfare transport to be transferred to the Local Health Authority. Whilst it became their responsibility for the ambulance service, there was a clause in the Act allowing co-operation and agreements between them and the voluntary services. As a result of this co-operation between the Authorities, the Red Cross and St John Ambulance on 30 June, 1948, 733 ambulances were operating within the ambit of the National Health Service.

The Register of Ambulance Stations was also transferred to the Local Health Authorities, who in 1949 issued their first Government Publication, the Directory of Ambulance Control Centres in England, Wales and Scotland.

Following this in the early 50s, Ford of Britain were asked by the Ministry of Defence to submit a four-wheel drive military truck chassis cab to carry a range of bodies, amongst which was a four-stretcher ambulance.

In 1950 Dennis Brothers designed and produced their A.V.

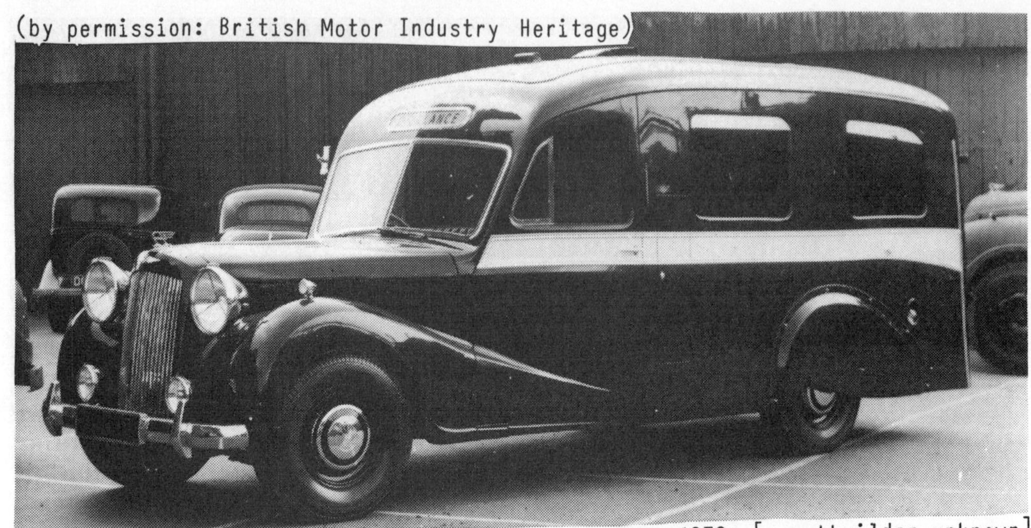

Austin Princess ambulance, 1950s [coachbuilder unknown]

Series of ambulance chassis, this model being specially designed to meet the requirements of ambulance operation. It had a special chassis frame and rear suspension, enabling a very low floor height to be provided to give easy loading and unloading of stretcher patients. Production extended into the 1960s.

Ford special military ambulance, 1952 [Four wheel drive chassis]

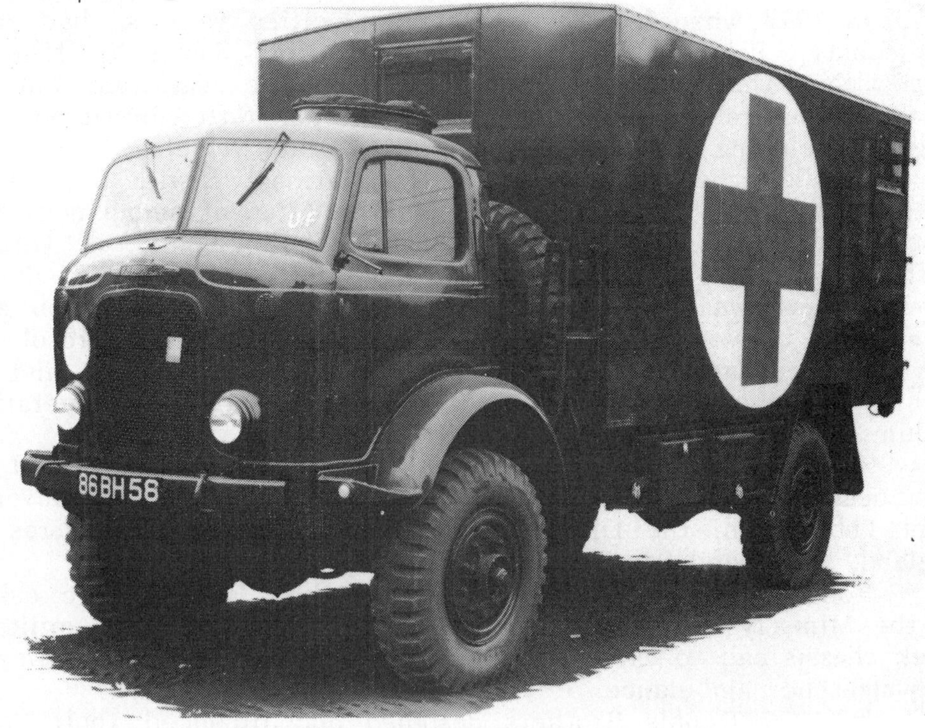

After five operational years of the National Health Service, there was a tendency for the St John and Red Cross voluntary services of ambulances to withdraw from the Service.

At the end of the first six months of the same year, 1953, miles of operational duties performed by the Central Ambulance Service of London with the County Council amounted to about 300,000, carrying 14,092 patients in the 30 ambulances involved.

In 1948 one of the popular body builders, Wadham Brothers (later to become Wadham Stringer (Coachbuilders) Ltd, after their merger with Stringers) made their appearance at the Commercial Motor Show at Earl's Court, displaying their bodies of buses, coaches and ambulances. At that time Morris and Austin were among the largest suppliers of ambulances for civil use, based on their standard van models which were of high production levels and therefore having the advantage in unit cost over Dennis, Daimler and other small production vehicle manufacturers.

In 1949 Wadham was appointed ambulance body supplier to Morris Commercial Cars Ltd., who were, effectively, the sole suppliers to the District Hospitals: besides this appointment the company was already building ambulances for St John Ambulance and the British Red Cross organisations.

With the advance made in the motor and commercial vehicle industries, especially in light and medium range vans, ambulances could be produced in three ways –

1. Complete ambulance body, designed, built and mounted on a vehicle chassis specially designed, or on a standard design of chassis completely modified for ambulance operation.

Austin 1 ton multi-fuel 4x4 military ambulance for 4 stretchers, 1962

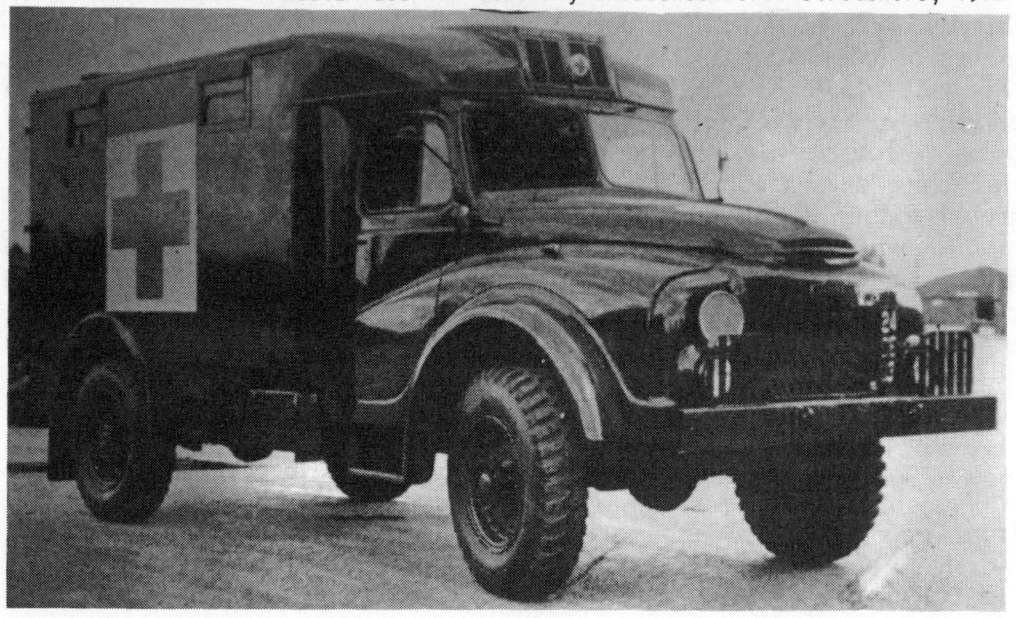

2. Complete ambulance bodies designed, built and mounted on a standard commercial manufactured van chassis front end, chassis cab or chassis cowl versions.
3. Conversions of standard manufactured van models.

In the 1950s the British Red Cross Society was using ambulances designed primarily to carry one stretcher, with provision for 3 or 4 sitting cases: if a second stretcher was required, then the seat on the offside could be lowered to allow for this. The ambulance was well ventilated, clean air being draw in via ducting, cold or hot as desired, the temperature being controlled by the nurse or attendant. Beneath the floor was a stainless steel container, well ventilated, in which was a bed pan and a urine bottle, access being by trap in the floor. Underneath an outlet was constructed in the form of a tunnel, so that the whole utensil and bottle could be drawn out from the outside of the ambulance. Clean water was provided for drinking in a glass stoppered bottle, housed in a locker: individual throw-away drinking cartons were used. Locker equipment was provided to house spare stretchers, blankets and other essential equipment. Last of all, there was a small surgery with a sink and running water, towel, etc., in a corner of the body. Another standardised type for the Society had a longer wheelbase and could carry 4 stretcher and 4 sitting cases or, alternatively, two stretcher and 8 sitting cases, or 12 sitting cases.

A coachbuilder, well-known for its quality products, was Vanden Plas who built high class ambulance bodies from 1959 to 1962 on the Austin Princess (A125) chassis and also supplied a 4 litre model chassis themselves to specialised coachbuilders.

Around the early 60s Dennis Brothers, in conjunction with Karrier Motors, Ltd., produced an ambulance to fill the requirements of easy access. The chassis was built by Karrier and was of the well-known Karrier/Commer 'Walk Thru' type of the 1½ton van chassis with choice of petrol or diesel engines, Dennis being responsible for the design and construction of the ambulance body. At this time several body builders were producing quite a number of styled ambulance bodies. Two of them, Wadham Stringer and Dormobile were converting Morris Commercial and Austin vans into ambulances, as well as building bodies and mounting them on van chassis front end versions, including Bedford, Ford and, later, B.M.C. Other builders started designing and constructing such bodies, including Pilcher-Greene, Hanlon and Lomas.

Wadham Stringer was becoming one of the largest builders of ambulance bodies in Britain. From 1963 they were either converting standard commercial medium range vans or mounting ambulance bodies onto specially built and prepared chassis and standard chassis front end versions, such as the Austin models 'FG' and 'LD5W'; Morris Commercial 'J2-M16' and 'J2'; later B.M.C. model '250JU'; Land Rover long wheelbase model; Ford Transit models 130, 160

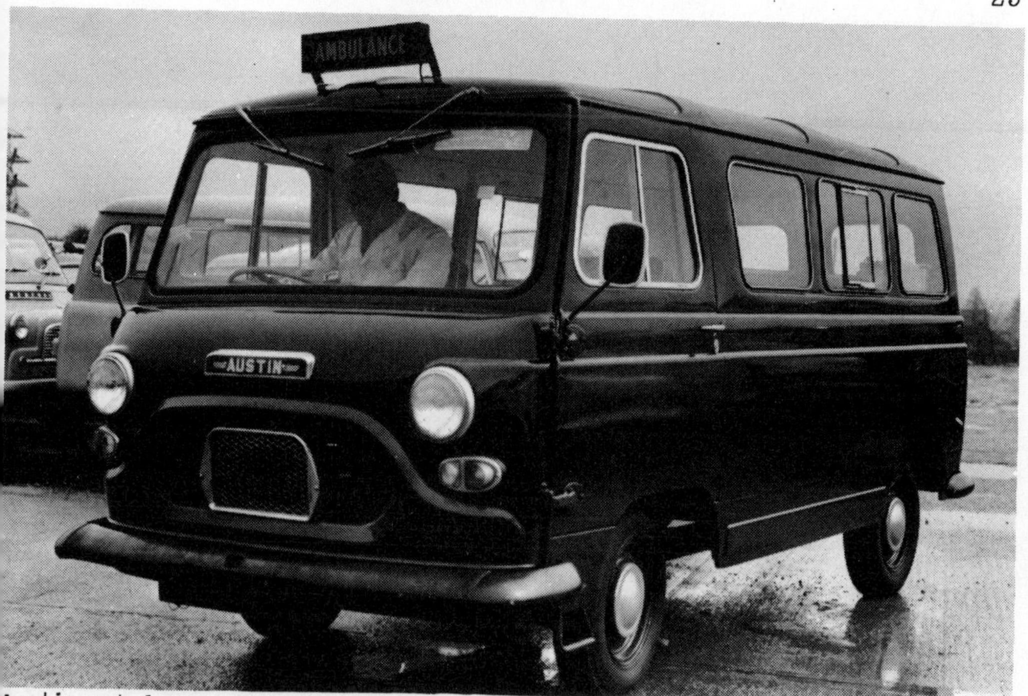

Austin ambulance with Dormobile body, 1965

and 175; Bedford 'CF' range models 280, 340 and 350; Leyland/ Morris 'Sherpa' (now Freight/Rover 'Sherpa') and Volkswagen model LT28. Special ambulance chassis for better comfort, ride and handling were introduced from British Leyland model 'FG'; Ford Transit model 160; Range Rover; and Bedford 'CF' range models 280 and 350.

The Royal Army Medical Corps obtained their own ambulances through the motor industry. They were searching for a small ambulance, go anywhere type, with accommodation for two and four stretcher cases. As a result of the success of the Land Rover, a four wheel drive machine already with the British Army, the Land Rover Company submitted an ambulance body by Marshalls of Cambridge, mounted on their Land Rover 2.77 metre wheelbase. It proved successful and was adopted. Later, Austin (B.M.C.) built and developed a four wheel drive version of their normal truck chassis with an ambulance body by Mann-Egerton of Norwich and submitted it to the military establishment for test and assessment. It had room for four stretcher cases, or two stretcher and four sitting cases, or 8 sitting cases.

The civilian outlets now depended upon the Local Health Authorities in the city and the county ambulance services, but there were many areas where the State service was inadequate and had to be supplemented by St John Ambulance Brigades and, at

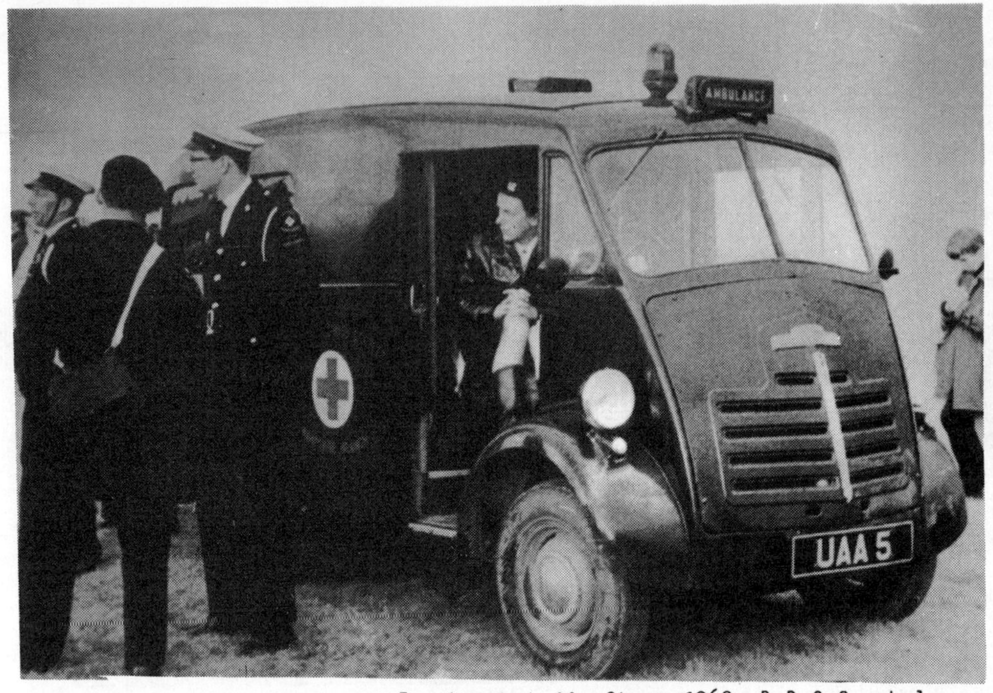

Farnborough Air Show, 1968   B R C S ambulance

times, the local British Red Cross. The two voluntary units were on
most occasions represented at sporting events or at demonstrations.
     From the earliest days the ambulance had been sent to the
disinfecting station only after infectious cases had been carried.
The responsibility is that of the Medical Officer of Health for the
particular area to ensure that ambulances are properly disinfected
after the conveyance of suspect patients. However, it was considered by the medical authorities that all ambulances should be
disinfected as a matter of routine after each journey or visit to a
hospital: so, after considerable investigation, a firm of chemists
produced a powerful new germicide that could be sprayed around
inside the ambulance. This particular disinfectant was non-
poisonous, non-caustic, non-irritant, non-staining, and was given a
pleasant odour. The inside of each ambulance in the British Red
Cross and St John Ambulance fleets is sprayed after carrying
patients, as are the National Health Service vehicles.
     Body construction had made rapid progress from the pre-1914
days of the horse-drawn ambulance with its canvas tilt and wooden
body. The first step had been to improve the ride of the wagon by
providing softer springs in the suspension and better fitting canvas
tilts to eliminate draughts, but still giving some sort of ventilation.
Improvements were made on motorised units; from wood frame and
treated stretched canvas covering and tongued and grooved wooden
'huts' to wooden framing and treated plywood panelling, painted

and varnished. Then came steel motor bodies to give new strength to the ambulance body: first it was sheet steel panels on hardwood framing, then light steel sectioned framing with thin sheet steel panelling. Both of these latter were internally panelled with treated plywood or hardboard and painted.

Then came the need to lighten the body for steel structure with the additional equipment being installed made the ambulance heavy and consequently demanded more power from the engine. The lightened body structure was of either hardwood framing reinforced at the joints with plates and brackets or aluminium top hat section framing, both with sheet aluminium panelling. Development of small engines with high horsepower, combined with lightweight bodies produced an acceptable ambulance in which the maximum equipment required could be installed without sacrificing patient capacity. This was fine, except for corrosion, which entailed specially treating the body before painting.

Then came the age of plastics and the motor body manufacturers took advantage of it. Glass fibre reinforced plastic (GRP) was introduced, formed into panels and fixed to either a hardwood or a light steel section frame. These glass fibre bodies had numerous advantages – they were light, strong, proof against

Interior Ford Model 7V ambulance, 1946 (by permission of Essex Ambulance Service)

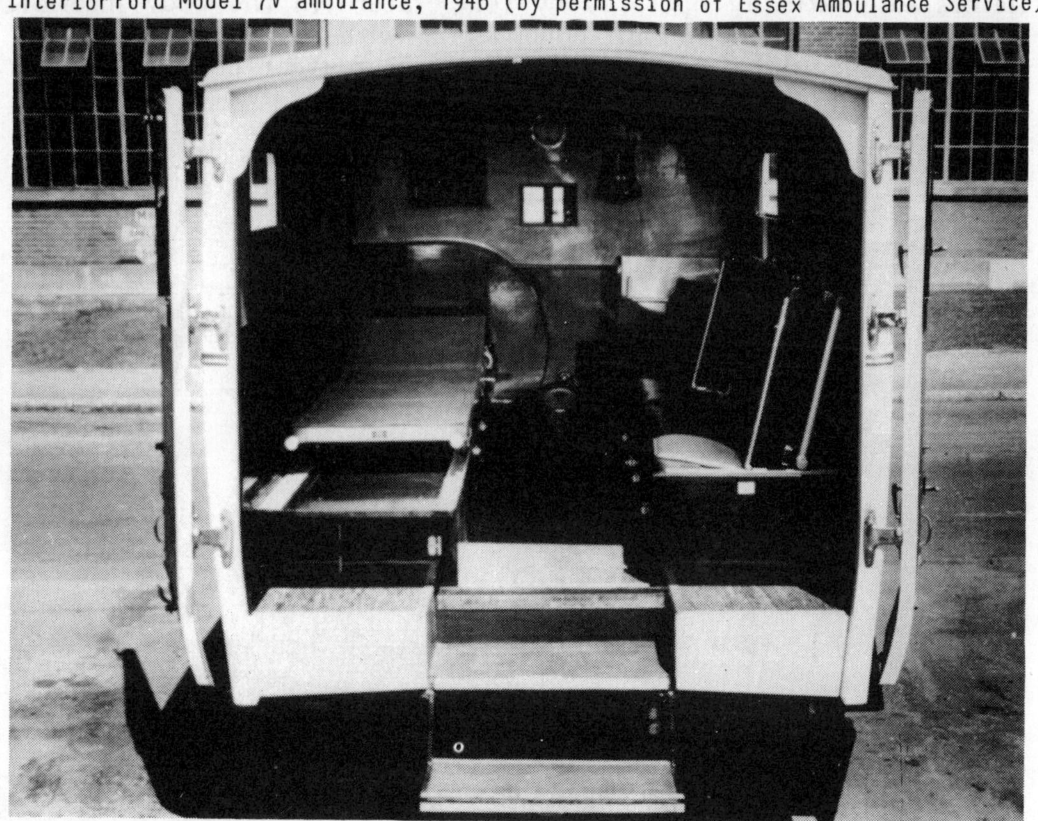

corrosion, requiring little or no maintenance, and repairs could be carried out quite easily on any part without having to replace whole body panels or parts by cutting and welding. A further feature that meant a great deal to the Local Health Authorities was the plastic which could be self-coloured, so there was no need for re-painting to keep appearance in good order, and cleaning was easier, an essential feature towards better hygiene. Another advantage became apparent when the whole body, even the framing, was constructed from GRP, although metal reinforcements had to be inserted to attach units or equipment and the chassis mountings.

Interior finishing had also progressed from no fitted interior panelling to plywood panels, then to hardboard type covered with a plastic surface, again self-coloured and easy to clean. Trimmings improved with either anodized or polished aluminium waist line strips with coloured plastic inserts, a more advanced method especially for interior use was chrome plated plastic strips.

Floors improved from bare wooden boards, which had to be constantly scrubbed clean, to thick treated plywood covered with good quality linoleum or Vinyl, both edged and sealed.

Ventilation problems were overcome by the installation of ventilators in the roof with hit and miss grills inside, also ventilators automatically operated by temperature in the body interior, opening windows and full air conditioning with recirculation units.

We seem to have almost reached the perfect body shell - or have we?

Interior of Austin ambulance with Dormobile body, 1965

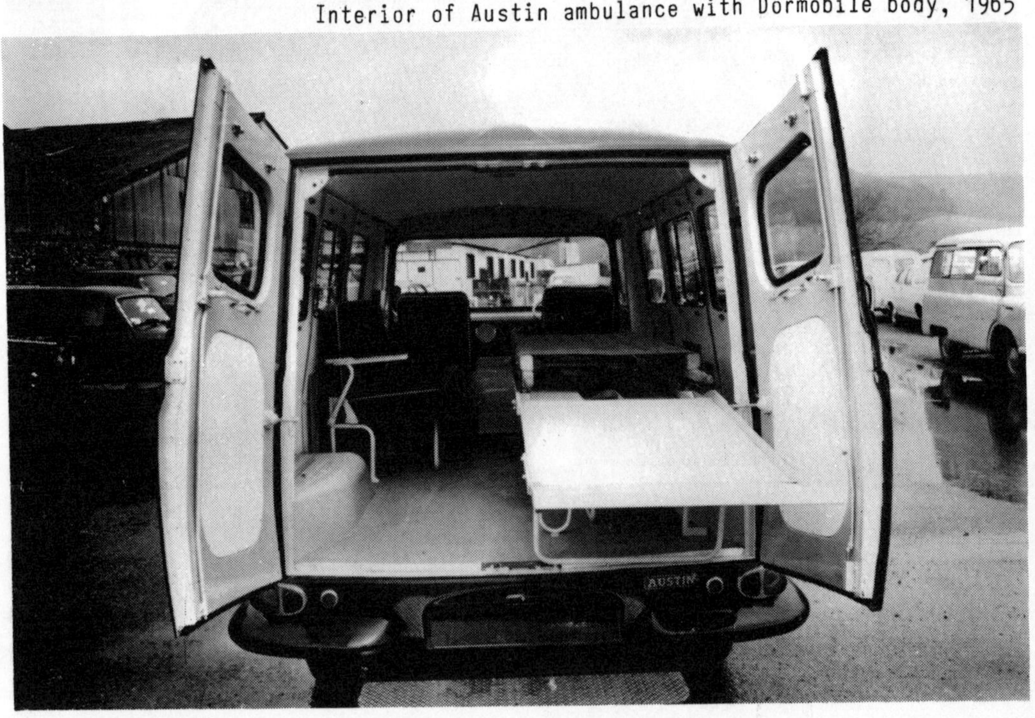

What about the interior? There is still a lot to be done to really give comfort and be able to provide better attention to the patients.

Many features of ambulances supplied in the past to the two voluntary organisations were primitive and somewhat crude by today's standards. The paint and varnished bodies had to be leathered off after a wet journey, as the rain left indelible marks on the paintwork, and materials used, while of good quality, were not easily kept clean. But then an ambulance was only a vehicle needed to carry sick, injured and wounded people to a hospital, not as today, almost like a travelling hospital in itself. With the equipment carried in the latest ambulances, the seriously ill patient stands a better chance of reaching the destination alive and of recovery.

Designs of stretchers has somewhat improved over the years; from the rough canvas or blanket material, two wooden poles and spreaders to the present comfortable stretcher trolley which, when placed on the stretcher rack after the patient has been wheeled into the ambulance, can be used as a temporary hospital bed. A turn-over type seat/stretcher rack, comprising a full bench type seat with cushions the structure of which is arranged to rotate and expose a full-length stretcher rack is provided in the modern ambulance.

Bench type seats are provided with backrests and folding armrests, double and single seats all with foam filled cushions and squabs for the comfort of sitting patients. Lightweight folding stretchers are still available to supplement the standard stretcher equipment, and stowed under the standard stretcher racks. Improved stowage and storage has been introduced. Partitions between the driver's compartment and the patients were fitted: some were full height and width with a sliding communication window in one half, while a door was installed in the other half. Other partitions were only part way up the height of the interior. Decency panels were fitted in front of seats near to entrances and exits.

Improvements in equipment were far reaching from almost nothing to first class equipment capable of taking care of almost any situation or emergency en route, from the birth of a child to a blood transfusion.

In the present day ambulance equipment includes quite a formidable assortment, some of which are listed below. [This equipment does not apply to any one particular ambulance]:

Vacuum flask in special holder
Portable first aid box
Water bottle with glass
Trolley mounted plasma bottle holder
Portable incubator supply point
Piped oxygen

Carry chair
Resuscitator
Spinal board
Orthopaedic stretcher
Direct oxygen supply to twin flowmeters from static cylinder, with additional Ambu Kompact set portable resuscitator
Portable aspirator
Inflatable splints and Kramer splints
'Vitalograph' resuscitator and intubation kit
Double infusion bottle holder and extension to 1346mm
Stretcher trolley, incorporating the posture drainage position, head/back rest adjustment with guard rails, pulling handles, recessed mattress, two-position locking device and telescopic loading handles

Below is the equipment installed in an ambulance, irrespective of the list above. Whilst all are available, not every ambulance has every item –

Full width folding rear step
Roof ventilators, manual and electrically operated extractors
Two external rear mirrors
Dual windshield wipers
Cab heater
Automatic safety belts fitted for driver's and nearside passenger's use
Four ambulance compartment interior lights, with switches inside rear entrance. Some installations provide for switches in the driver's compartment. The lights are fitted in each corner of the ambulance compartment at roof height.
Grab handles fitted each side of the ambulance interior above the side windows
Night-driving blind for driver (concertina type)
Manually operated windshield washer
Lockers fitted in convenient locations, including medical locker for drugs and medicines
Fire extinguishers in driver's cab
Fuel cut-off valve fitted in the fuel line, capable of being operated from outside
Battery isolation switch in driver's cab
Roof beacon and repeaters
Ambulance compartment heater
Twin tone horns
Radio accommodation
Loading lights
Warning tapes on sides and at the rear of the body
Tropical roof panels
Head bumper pads over rear entrance
Twin sun visors
Fog and spot lights and switches in driver's compartment
Illuminated 'AMBULANCE' sign in front at roof height

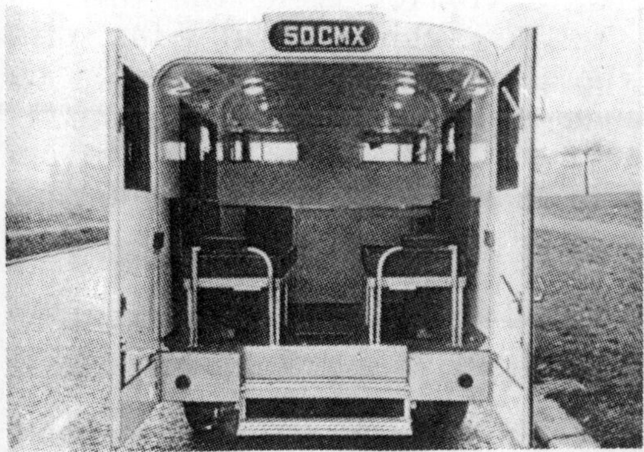

Dennis Model A.V. series ambulance:
interior

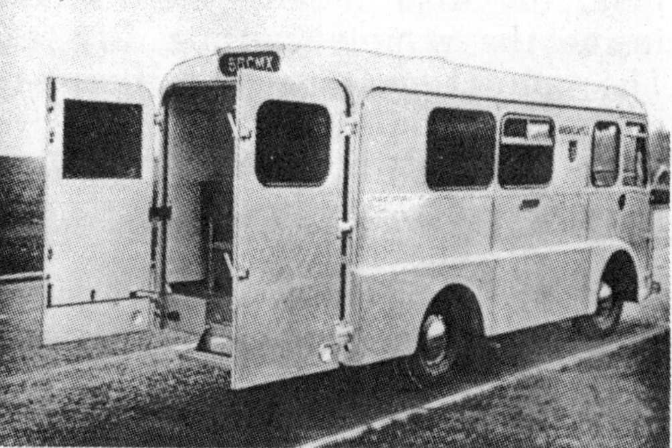

Dennis Model A.V. series ambulance:
rear view

Reviewing the progress made over the years to improve the ambulance vehicle, there still seems a great deal to be done to find a machine as the ideal conveyance of the sick and injured.

The ambulance is the most important vehicle of any service, for the ride characteristics can seriously affect the suffering and even the chances of recovery of a seriously ill or injured patient: it is therefore essential to get the suspension right.
The success of any suspension depends upon the proper balance between the springs (coil or leaf), shock absorbers and tyres. It must be designed to give the correct periodicity for both front and rear and to harmonise with no front pitching or soft spongy ride, which can result in patients suffering from seasickness.

A satisfactory body and layout has been achieved, coming from suggestions and ideas from the London Ambulance Service operational staff and other professionals throughout the country. Unfortunately, however, no satisfactory vehicle chassis has been designed. London Ambulance bought a number of Daimler ambulances based on the D27 car chassis, which was quite a good vehicle, but went out of production in the mid-fifties.

We are left with an ambulance chassis modified in the suspension and the fitting of low pressure tyres, the base having been primarily designed for the carriage of goods.

A working party was set up - one of many over the years - to investigate the requirements of an ambulance vehicle and recommend a suitable specification. Their findings suggested that a suitable vehicle would have - front-wheel drive to ensure a low floor, independent suspension on all four wheels to assist in giving a good ride; a powerful engine to ensure smoothness and reasonable gradeability at reasonable speed; a low floor without sacrificing belly clearance to negotiate unmade roads; and an automatic transmission for smooth take-off and less driver fatigue. All this except the type of the vehicle; normal control, forward control or semi-forward control.

The advantage of a fully forward control is in the driver's forward vision of the road close to his vehicle, while the disadvantage is in the protrusion of the engine and gearbox into the driver's cab, restricting easy entrance and exit from his compartment. It also means that servicing has to be carried out from inside the vehicle causing difficulty in maintaining a clean interior. The advantages of the normal control is the straight through entrance and exit from the driver's compartment and easy serving from outside the vehicle. However, it does have the disadvantage that the driver's forward vision of the road is not close to the front of his vehicle and is therefore limited. The semi-forward control, the compromise version, has the advantage of reasonable forward vision, while the intrusion of the engine inside the driver's compartment is small, so easy entrance and exit can be achieved. Servicing can be carried out outside the ambulance by the removal of the front grille and panel and the ample opening provided by the short bonnet. This design is the one most commonly used at the present time.

The G.L.C. contributed towards research on the subject of a suitable chassis to find if a vehicle earlier described as being towards the ideal could be produced at reasonable cost. The only way this can be done is for a single manufacturer to design such a vehicle and adopt the same design for his general commercial programme, even if it were one model with economical production quantity. To produce a special vehicle to the ideal specification would involve very high production costs.

This was confirmed when Dennis Brothers set about designing a special purpose-built ambulance chassis around the findings of a Home Office working party. It featured a front-wheel drive, leaving an exceptionally low rear entrance; powered by the Jaguar petrol engine for both quietness and smooth running with a full automatic transmission, and a low floor level – everything that was required! Unfortunately and regretably the venture was 'killed off' due to high production costs.

Nevertheless, such commercial vehicle manufacturers as Bedford and Ford operate a Special Vehicle Operations Department to build special versions and conversions of the 'CF' and the Transit ranges.

London Ambulance Service had been operating B.M.C., model L.D. chassis, for ambulances since 1965, but this model was superseded by the manufacturer with a new chassis not really suiting ambulance work. The Service changed to Bedford and Ford with passable results, but these models have been fitted with special features to endeavour to meet working requirements – which would not suit the military side of ambulance transport where high belly clearances, approach and departure angles are needed.

The L.C.C. Supplies Department did pioneer the production of a fibreglass ambulance body that was constructed by the Department until 1965, when they ceased. Wadham Brothers took over the work and continued to produce this type of body to the Council's specification.

Probably the best solution is independent suspension, both front and rear, with a hydraulic levelling device, but even this scheme could present a cost penalty. Efficient lighting, internally and externally is necessary: internal to assist the attendant or nurse to see to fulfill their duties to the patient en route, externally for the driver's visibility during the hours of darkness or other weather conditions. Adequate lighting should be available to load and unload the patient, especially during dull weather and after dark. It is necessary that battery capacity and alternator or generator output is sufficient to give power and charging facilities to fulfil the requirements of the ambulance or welfare vehicle's additional electrical equipment and that of the medical equipment installed. Performance is another feature of importance to successful operation. The ambulance must be able to speed along and to negotiate reasonable gradients at a reasonable speed (it is no good just climbing gradients in bottom gear at ten miles per hour!), the essential factor is speed/gradient. Speed and safety with reliability are essential to operate an efficient service.

Sufficient engine power is required with the correctly selected transmission and rear axle ratios to give a good vehicle performance. Automatic tranmissions have become available on some manufacturers' chassis and offer a smoother ride with less driver fatigue.

Martin Walter ambulance body on B.M.C. "FG" chassis, 1966

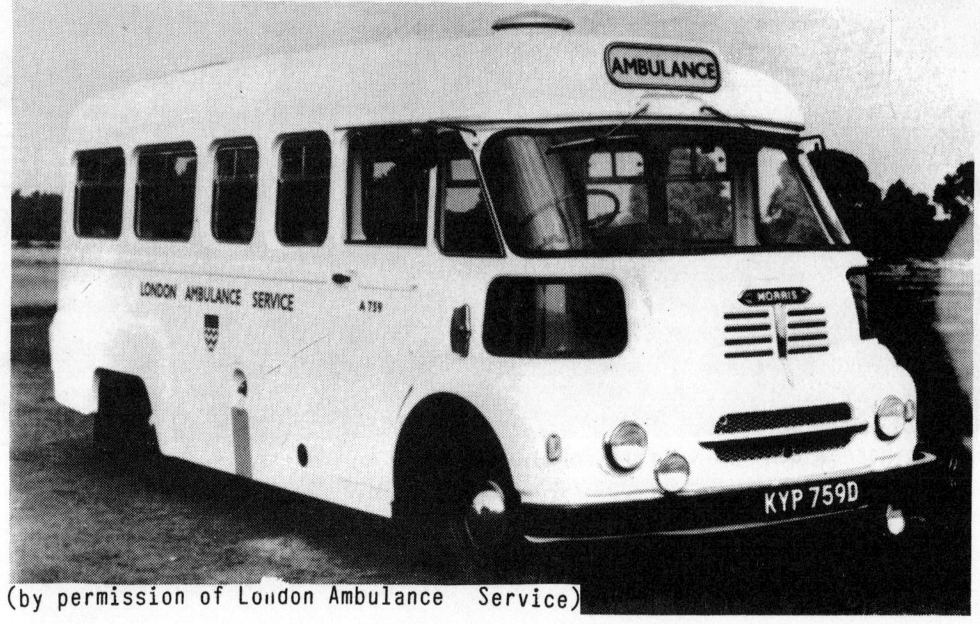

(by permission of London Ambulance Service)

Noise insulation is another feature needed both inside and out: in the engine compartment, underneath the body and the chassis. A feature not often considered in vehicles is the location of the exhaust pipe, which should be placed, within regulation limits, in positions where fumes cannot enter the body even when there is a fault in the system and repairs have to be made.

Perhaps some day a vehicle manufacturer may produce the ideal chassis, but once more, unless reasonable quantities can be produced, the cost will remain high.

The total patient carrying fleet of the London Ambulance Service, now under the National Health Service, was, in 1973 – 968 ambulances and sitting case vehicles, housed at 78 stations made up of 30 large stations with 20 to 60 vehicles, both stretcher ambulances and sitting case ambulances, and 48 small stations with up to 6 stretcher ambulances engaged primarily on emergency work. Generally vehicles are replaced every 7 years or on completion of 100,000 miles, but each vehicle is judged according to its individual condition before any decision is reached.

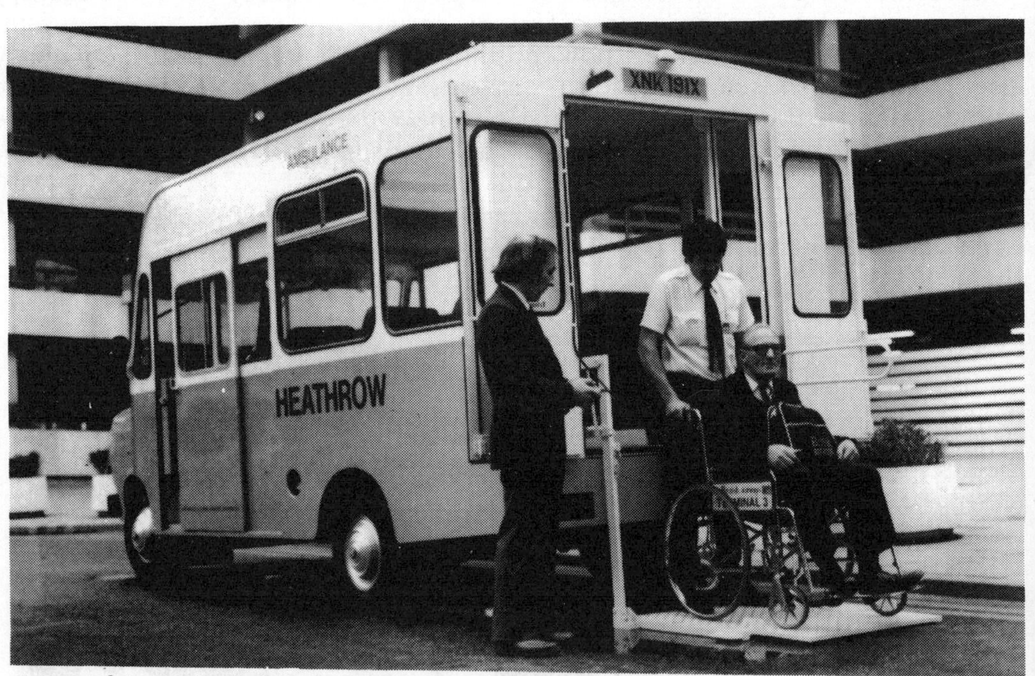

Hawson-Garner body on welfare ambulance, 1980s

Welfare Vehicles

Welfare Authorities have the problem of moving elderly and disabled people in comfort and safety to hospitals for their periodic visits, to social events and for general welfare duties. It needs a fleet of specialised vehicles, such as ambulances and properly prepared buses for the carriage of the elderly and the disabled.

Using virtually the same basic vehicle as for the general ambulances, special bodies were designed and made available to the Welfare Authorities to meet the demand for vehicles to cope with the transport of patients, including invalids confined to wheelchairs.

For the latter, tail lifts, manually or electro-hydraulically operated, were provided to help in their loading and unloading.

The body construction was similar to the general ambulance; aluminium section framing and panelling, or light section steel framing and glass fibre reinforced plastic panelling, etc.

Special interior features were quick lock wheelchair clamps and/or wheelchair restraint straps to secure wheelchairs to the special rails inserted into the compartment floor of the vehicle. Special seat legs with fixings that can also be pushed into the same floor rails when, with a turn of the legs, the seat becomes secured to the floor. Single and double passenger seats, safety harness, head-rests and folding armrests are among the other items of equipment.

There are a number of welfare models being built by coachbuilders such as Hawson-Garner, Ltd., Dormobile, Ltd., B Walker, Son, Ltd., and Wadham Stringer(Coachbuilders), Ltd.

Each ambulance and bus body builder provides a set of standard interior layouts for seats, seat/stretcher and wheelchair accommodation, based on research of ambulance operators' and Local Authorities' requirements. Where standard layouts do not meet the needs, special layouts are drawn up and arranged to meet the accommodation requested.

With the special seat slide tracks inserted in the floor, it does not become hard to replace one, or even a number, of seats for a stretcher rack or a wheelchair.

However, there is still a lot more room for improvement.

Vehicle Specifications

This chapter describes many of the ambulance and welfare vehicles in 3 sections -
Section 1: Construction and specifications of ambulance bodies, including the interior layouts.
Section 2: Construction and specifications of welfare vehicle bodies, including the interior layouts.
Section 3: Specifications of the basic motor vehicles and chassis used for ambulances and welfare vehicles.

SECTION ONE
The following descriptions are those taken from a few well-known coachbuilders to show the typical construction of ambulance bodies made during this century. Some of the other coachbuilders' bodies are similar in construction with small differences in styling.

To be competitive today, bodies from any coachbuilder should depend on standardisation of panelling and body framing, roofs and windows, and basically should be able to be mounted on most commercial van-type chassis. There are, of course, the individual special ambulances required by various organisations and variations in wheelbases and rear overhangs, which can be taken care of by inserting sections to cater for the differences.

It is not possible to take the specifications of all coach-builders engaged in manufacturing ambulance bodies without creating a volume of data that would become repetitive. Therefore the body constructions and specifications are generalised and could be used by any body builder.

The construction of the body shell includes interior panelling, doors, windows, roofing and rear entrances.

Body Shell Construction Specification No. C1 (1914-18)
The base of the body was similar to that of a flat platform truck with sides, front board and tailboard.
Framing   Hardwood vertical strips fixed to the top of the sides with a horizontal top rail along the sides of the body at roof height forming two side frames.

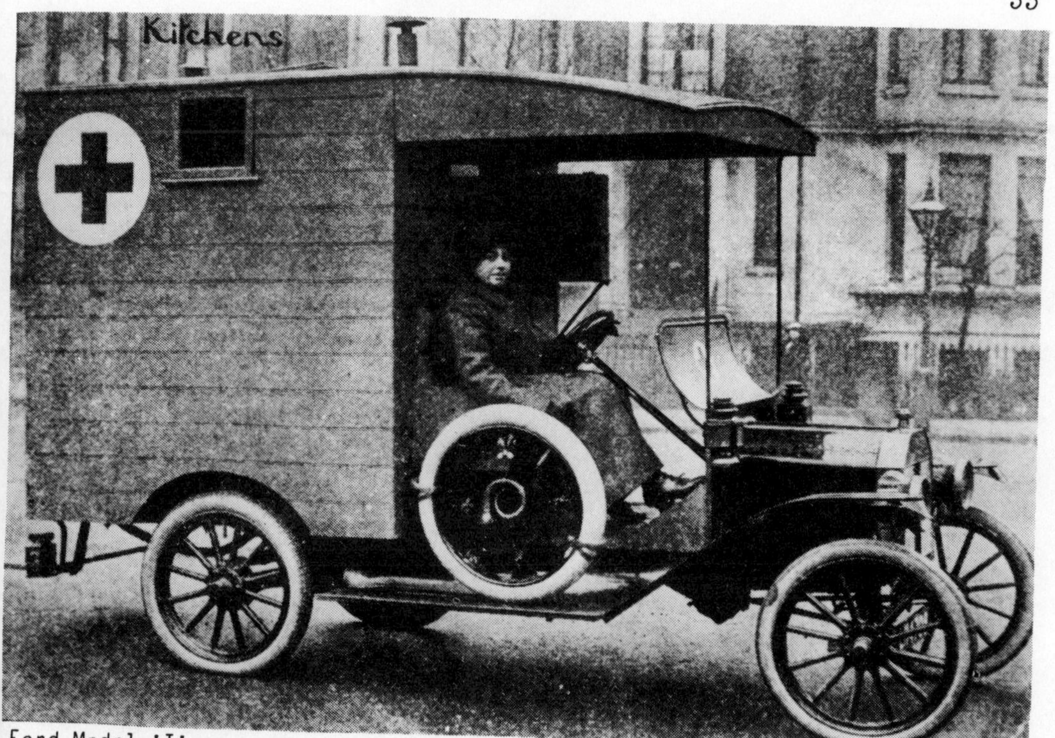

Ford Model 'T'

External panelling　Stretched canvas fixed to side frames and treated for weather proofing.

Roof　Wooden formers transversely across the top of the side frames. Stretched canvas covering fixed to the roof formers and treated for weather proofing.

Floor　Plain wood. No covering.

Doors　No rear doors. Canvas curtains, rolled up to roof level when not in use.

<u>Body Shell Construction Specification No. C2</u>

Early type used during the latter part of the war for civilians.

Framing　Hardwood with the corners reinforced with thin triangular iron plates and corner brackets. Treated before panelling.

External panelling　Plywood panels fixed to framing and floor. Treated before painting.

Roof　Plain top of plywood, treated for weather proofing and fitted with ventilator.

Floor　Thick plywood fixed to body side runner and transverse beams. Covered with good quality linoleum.

Doors　Two hinged rear doors.

Windows　Two each side above the waist line. One in each rear door.

Body Shell Construction Specification No. C3

This is the body specification for the Dennis special ambulance built in 1915.

Framing   Best selected ash wood, well seasoned and knot free. Joints tenoned and mortised and accurately fitted together with white lead. Mild steel plates fitted at the joints where necessary to ensure rigidity.

 External panelling   Selected Honduras mahogany and canary white wood lined with canvas and painted.

Roof and canopy   Roofing or 3-ply birch venesta in one piece and covered with the best canvas unjointed and treated for weather proofing. The canopy projects in front of the dash, fitted with a water cornice.

Floor   19.05mm (.75 inch) thick birch wood, rabetted together and screwed down and brass edged. The whole covered in linoleum.

Interior panelling   All of the best 3-ply venesta white wood. Treated before painting.

Doors   Two hinged rear doors to open across the full width of the body.

Windows   One at each side and one at the rear hinged in the centre to allow the top half to drop inwards as required. Sliding window at the front behind the driver. No windows in the rear doors.

Step   At the rear, arranged to fold up when not in use; the tread covered in linoleum and brass edged.

Body Shell Construction Specification No. C4 (1948 to 1952)

This is the body construction by Barker & Co. (Coachbuilders) Ltd. for the Daimler ambulance (Model D27 chassis) –

Framing   Ash wood, reinforced with plywood and steel at the joints where necessary. Treated before panelling.

Exterior panelling   Aluminium sheets. Treated before painting.

Roof   Aluminium sheets. Treated before painting.

Floor   Exterior grade plywood. Driver's compartment covered with ribbed aluminium sheet. Ambulance compartment finished in Induroleum.

Interior panelling   In hardboard and covered with aluminium sheets.

Doors   Two full length rear.

Windows   Driver's compartment windows on winding mechanism. Two half-drop type windows are fitted either side and forward offside window is made to hinge inwards to form a means of emergency exit. All windows in driver's compartment toughened glass and all in the ambulance compartment in safety glass. Windshield split type with two side panels, toughened safety glass.

Step   Drop type – two step central single width step.

Body Shell Construction Specification No. C5 (1965 to 1980s)

Complete bodywork of double skinned colour impregnated moulded glassfibre reinforced plastic construction. Reinforced sections bonded in as necessary for securing fittings and equipment. Wheelboxes are of reinforced plastic construction.

Floor   From 16mm (0.62 inch) exterior grade bonded plywood covered with good quality linoleum.

Doors   Two hinged type at the rear.

Windows   In the driving compartment on winding mechanism in the doors. Large double windows, forward section of which incoporates top-half sliding units in ambulance compartment. Fixed windows in rear doors. Half-sliding communication window in the partition between the driver and the ambulance compartment and fixed window in the partition door. Two piece wrapped-round windshield. Clear double 'Shadowlite' coloured safety glass in ambulance compartment windows.

Step   Full width step well and additional drop-out step at the rear entrance.

Body Shell Construction Specification No. C6 (1965)

Framing   Selected hardwood, joints synthetic resin glued and reinforced where necessary with mild steel plates and brackets. Treated before panelling.

Exterior panelling   In 18 s.w.g.thick aluminium sheets with joints sealed and covered with aluminium sections.

Floor   From 16mm (0.62 inch) thick exterior grade plywood resin bonded, covered with good quality linoleum.

Roof   Exterior in one piece glassfibre reinforced plastic construction with interior panel of 20 s.w.g.mild steel sheet.

Interior panelling   In plastic-faced hardboard with breather eyelets to stop between- panel condensation.

Doors   Two rear hinged.

Windows   In driving compartment on winding mechanism. Two large windows forward section, which incorporates top-half sliding units on both sides of body. Fixed windows in rear doors. Half sliding communication windows fitted in partition between driver and ambulance and a fixed window in the partition door. Clear safety glass for the driving compartment and the partition window, clear 'Shadowlite' coloured safety glass for the ambulance compartment.

Step   Full width step well and additional drop-out step fitted at rear entrance.

Body Shell Construction Specification No. C7 (1966)

Framing   Mild steel section, bolted, welded and rivetted together. Reinforced where necessary with gusset plates and brackets. Treated before panelling.

Exterior panelling   In 18 s.w.g. thick aluminium sheeting. All joints sealed and covered with aluminium sections.

Roof   One piece glassfibre reinforced plastic construction, with interior panelling of 22 s.w.g. mild steel sheet.

Floor   Supplied as part of the vehicle chassis, but extended at the rear. Covered with good quality linoleum.

Interior panelling   Good quality 3mm (0.12 inch) hardboard. Treated before painting.

Doors   Two hinged doors

Windows   One with top half sliding and one fixed in each side. One fixed in each rear door. Of toughened clear glass 4.7mm (0.18 inch) thick or coloured laminated safety glass.

Step   Double folding at the rear built into the skirt panel below the rear doors for easy access.

Body Shell Construction Specification No. C8 (1966)

The specification covers van body conversions only, therefore the actual con-struction of the body shell is as supplied by the vehicle manufacturers.

However, the following are additions and modifications carried out by the bodybuilder as part of the body shell –

Interior panelling   Sides below the waist lined with good quality painted hardboard. Window finishers of moulded plastic. Clip-on 'Furflex' finishers.

Windows   One half sliding windows and two fixed windows each side. All windows 4.7mm (0.18 inch) thick safety glass, coloured to suit operators' requirements. If coloured glazing is requested, then the rear door glass will be changed to suit.

Body Shell Construction Specification No. C9 (1976)

Framing   Folded light steel section, welded and bolted as necessary. Treated before panelling.

Exterior panelling   In 18 s.w.g. thick aluminium sheet. All joints sealed and lapped. Treated before finishing.

Roof   Exterior   –   one   piece   moulded   glassfibre   reinforced   plastic construction.

Floor   Thick 9mm (0.35 inch) exterior grade tropicalised plywood, covered with good quality Vinyl and sealed at the edges.

Interior panelling   Plastic faced hardboard. Thermal insulant between the inner and outer panels.

Doors   Two hinged rear.

Windows   One large each side of body, fixed in rear doors. Half sliding communication window in the partition between the driver's and ambulance compartments. Clear safety glass for the driver's cab and clear double 'Shadowlite' coloured safety glass for the ambulance.

Step   Single central folding rear.

Body Shell Construction Specification No. C10 (1980s)

Framing   Light steel section, welded together. Reinforced where necessary with gusset plates and brackets.

Exterior panelling   In glassfibre reinforced plastic.

Roof   In one piece moulded glassfibre reinforced plastic.

Floor   In resin bonded plywood covered with good quality linoleum.

Interior panelling   In glassfibre reinforced plastic.

Doors   Two rear hinged in glassfibre reinforced plastic with metal reinforcements for fittings.

Windows   Large double window units on both sides of the body with sliding units in both sections of the windows. Complete units arranged as an emergency exit   with glazing insert section with pull ring and notice of operation. Fixed windows in rear doors. All windows of safety glass, double 'Shadowlite' coloured for the ambulance compartment.

Step   Single folded step held by robust latch when closed at the rear, and centre step well.

The following 5 specifications show the type of ambulance body finish used -

Finish Specification No.F1

This is the specification for the Dennis ambulance of 1915 -

Interior   Sized and varnished.

Exterior   Body work is properly filled in, rubbed down and flattened, painted, lined and varnished in the best London coach style in colour selected.

Signs   Lettering, crests and coats-of-arms can be painted on body if so desired.

Finish Specification No. F2

Interior   Driver's compartment lined with cream impregnated panels. Ambulance compartment lined with white impregnated panels. Roof centre section left translucent giving maximum interior natural light. Lettering giving operation of the rear door locks.

Exterior   Impregnated single colour to customers' requirements. Wheels & bumpers left in factory finish.

Signs   Illuminated 'AMBULANCE' sign incorporated in the front of the roof or on the front and the rear of the roof as required.

Finish Specification No. F3

Interior   Cab and body sides and roof are painted in dust repellant multi-colour surfacing. Floor and rear wheelhouses painted with brown lino paint. Seat and stretcher frames in simulated hammer-finish synthetic enamel.

Exterior   In single colour synthetic enamel to customers' requirements. Wheels & bumpers in black. Lettering to customers' requirements.

Signs   Illuminated 'AMBULANCE' sign fitted to the front of the roof with switch adjacent to the driver. Word 'Ambulance' written each side of vehicle and across the rear doors to comply with H M Customs & Excise requirements for tax exemption, unless other lettering is required.

Finish Specification No. F4

For body shells constructed from glassfibre reinforced plastics both exterior and interior of body as Nos. C5 and C10 Body Shell Construction Specifications.

Interior   Single colour throughout.

Exterior   Single colour throughout. Wheels & bumpers left as chassis finish.

Signs   Illuminated 'AMBULANCE' sign incorporated in the front panel. Word 'Ambulance' written across the rear doors or at roof height at the rear when requested.

Finish Specification No. F5

This is the specification for the Daimler ambulance by Barker & Co. (Coachbuilders) Ltd. on chassis Model D27 -

Interior   Finish in super glossy surface in ivory coloured paint.

Exterior   Finish in zinc chromate primer. Colour at customers' request.

Signs   'AMBULANCE' sign built into roof above windshield.

Ambulance Body Specifications

Note: Specifications 1 – 4 are for standard van conversons: 5 to 16 are for full ambulance bodies fitted to van chassis cab, chassis front end and chassis cowl versions also specially designed ambulance chassis.

Body Specification No. 1

Four standard interior layouts for the seats and the stretchers –

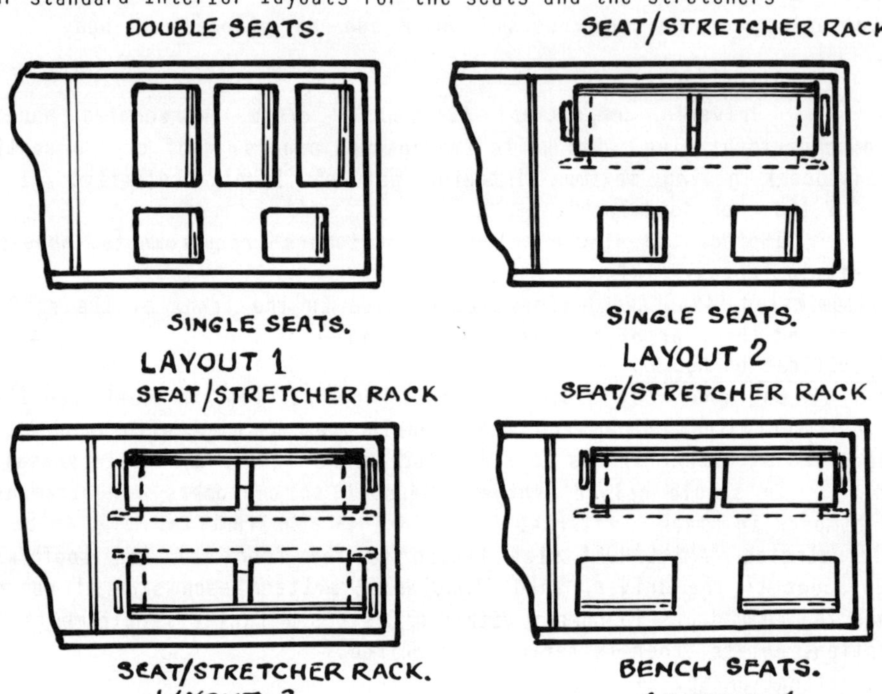

1. 3 forward facing double seats with folding backrests on the offside. The backrests fold forward onto the seat cushions and allow the stretcher rack to hinge down from the body side. 2 forward facing single seats on the nearside. A folding stretcher supplied which, when not in use, may be stowed at the offside cant rail.
Accommodation – 8 sitting cases, or 2 sitting cases and 1 stretcher case.
2. Turnover seat/stretcher rack fitted to offside. This comprises a full-length bench seat for up to 5 people, with cushions; structure arranged to rotate and expose full-length stretcher rack. 2 forward facing single seats fitted on nearside. A folding stretcher supplied which, when not in use, may be stowed beneath the turnover seat. Accommodation – 7 sitting cases, or 2 sitting cases and 1 stretcher case.
3. Turnover seat/stretcher rack on both near- and off-sides. Accommodation – 10 sitting cases, or 5 sitting cases and 1 stretcher case, or 2 stretcher cases. Note: this layout is not suitable with side loading doors.
4. Turnover seat/stretcher rack fitted on the offside. 2 side facing bench type seats on the nearside. A folding stretcher which, when not in use, may be

stowed under the turnover seat. Accommodation - 9 sitting cases, or 4 sitting cases and 1 stretcher case.

Body Specification No. 2

4 standard interior layouts for the seats and stretchers -

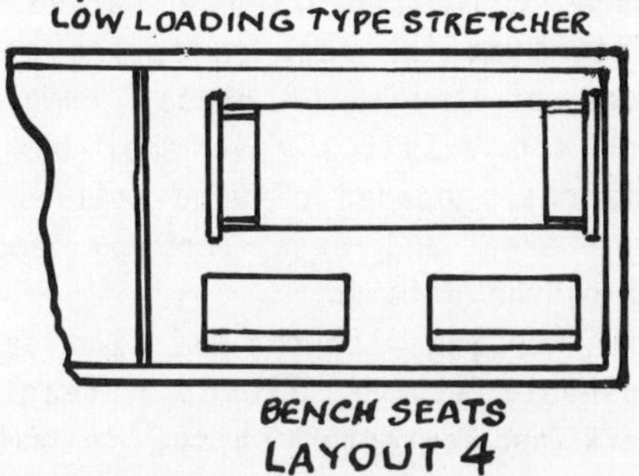

1. Layout similar to Specification No. 1, layout 2, except for accommodation - this layout is for 6 people on the full-length bench seat, and 3 forward facing single seats are fitted on the nearside. Accommodation - 9 sitting cases, or 3 sitting cases and 1 stretcher case.
2. Layout similar to Specification No. 1, layout 4, except for capacity - this layout is for 2 people on the full-length bench seat. Accommodation - 10 sitting cases, or 4 sitting cases and 1 stretcher case.
3. As for Specification No. 1, layout 1.
4. Low loading type stretcher on the offside. 2 bench type seats facing inwards on the nearside. Accommodation - 4 sitting cases and 1 stretcher case.

Body Specification No. 3

2 standard interior layouts for the seats and stretchers -

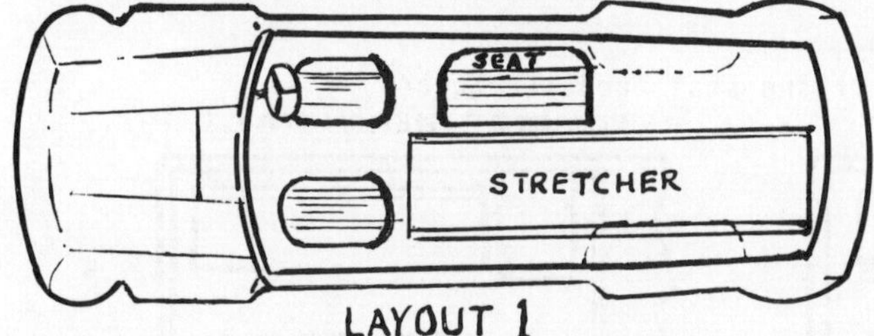

1. Attendant's seat fitted on offside behind driver's seat. Special trolley incorporating backrest adjustment fitted on nearside, complete with foam mattress with raised edges. Accommodation - Possible 1 sitting case as well as 1 stretcher case.
2. Full width bench seat behind the driver's seat. This is divided into 2 sections: the offside fixed for use by the attendant and the nearside folding down to form a level base for a stretcher. Stretcher rack of aluminium section fitted to nearside section of floor. Special stretcher with telescopic handles, white nylon coated canvas base, and recessed mattress provided. When not in use, folds transversely and is stowed in the rear behind the seats.

This specification is a conversion of a motorcar, the Austin 3 litre saloon. As the converson is exclusive to this particular car, the complete ambulance specification is -

General construction - existing bodywork above the guttering, rear boot assembly and the rear frame support panel are cut away to fit a new moulded glass reinforced plastic assembly incorporating a raised roof and extended rear section. Lift-up flap fitted at the rear on spring assistors and incorporating a large fixed window of toughened glass, complete with interior spring roll blind. Boot floor and existing rear seat box assembly finished level with the exterior grade resin bonded plywood covered with good quality linoleum, this forms a clear area and base for the ambulance equipment. Exhaust tail pipe is extended to the offside.

Finish - new interior finish in keeping with the existing car finish. Interior sides of rear lined with washable lining. Floor at rear covered with good quality linoleum. All new work and exterior white, to match existing basic motorcar finish.

'Ambulance' written on the rear in red letters. Lettering and fixed crests supplied by the Authorities. All doors and handles marked in accordance with the Ministry's recommendation.

Equipment - trolley mounted plasma bottle. First aid box in retaining tray on floor behind the attendant's seat. Vacuum flask. Illuminated 'AMBULANCE' sign incorporated in the front of the roof and wired through the side lamp circuit. Fluorescent interior illumination light. Automatic safety belts fitted to driver's and nearside attendant's seats. This is a typical specification for the conversion of large motorcars into small ambulances with one stretcher accommodation, usually used by small hospitals, nursing and convalescent homes, also private ambulance services.

Body Specification No. 4

This is a modern van conversion.

Two standard interior layouts for the seats and stretchers -

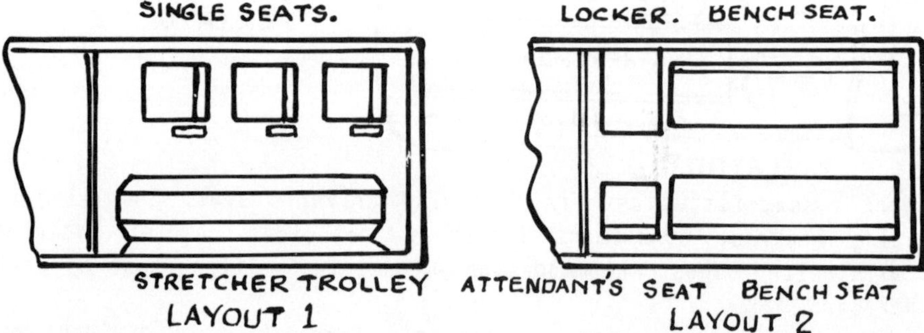

1. 3 forward facing single seats on the offside. Stretcher trolley on the nearside. Accommodation - 6 sitting cases, or 3 sitting cases and 1 stretcher case.

2. One seat facing attendant's seat and bench seat on nearside. Stowage locker behind the driver's seat with bench type seat on offisde. Accommodation - 10 sitting cases.

Body Specification No. 5
4 standard interior layouts for the seats and stretchers -

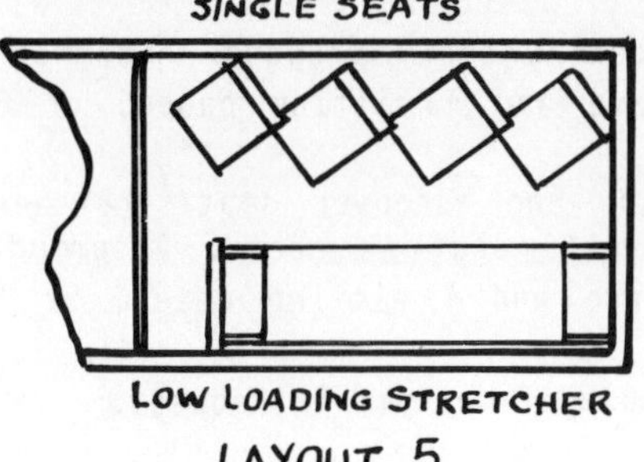

1. Turnover seat/stretcher rack fitted to nearside. Longitudinal bench seat fitted to offside. Accommodation - 8 sitting cases, or 4 sitting cases and 1 stretcher case.
2. Layout similar to Specification No. 1, layout 3, except for capacity, 6 people a side. Accommodation - 12 sitting cases, or 6 sitting cases and 1 stretcher case, or 2 stretcher cases.
3. 3 forward facing single seats on nearside. Turnover seat/stretcher, comprising bench seats for 6 sitting patients on offside. Accommodation - 9 sitting cases, or 3 sitting cases and 1 stretcher case.
4. 3 forward facing single seats on nearside. 3 double forward facing seats with backrests, which can be folded forward to take a stretcher rack on offside. Accommodation - 9 sitting cases, or 3 sitting cases and 1 stretcher case.

Body Specification No. 6
6 standard interior layouts for the seats and stretchers -

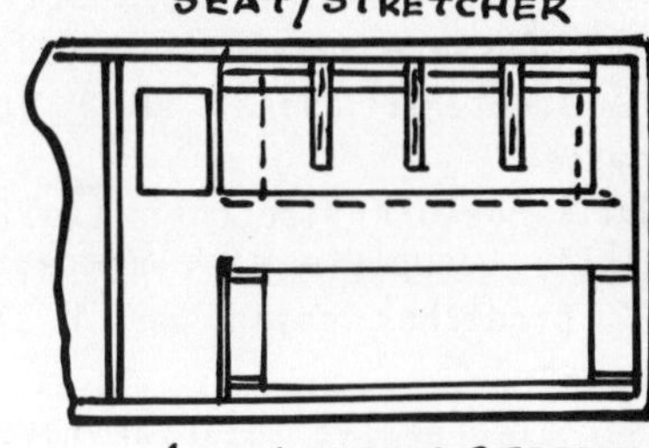

4 of these layouts, 1 to 4 are as for Specification No. 5, layouts 1,2,3, and 4. The other layouts are -
5. Low loading type stretcher gear on nearside, mounted on a locker and incorporating a self-elevating foam bed. 4 single echelon seats on offside, one fixed alloy stretcher. Accommodation - 4 sitting cases and 1 stretcher case.

6. Low loading type stretcher gear on nearside mounted on a locker and with a self-elevating bed. Turnover seat/stretcher rack with 3 folding armrests and mounted on a locker on offside. Attendant's seat in front offside corner. One fixed and one folding light alloy stretcher. Accommodation - 1 stretcher case and 3 sitting cases, or 2 stretcher cases.

Body Specification No. 7

A standard interior layout for the seats and stretchers -

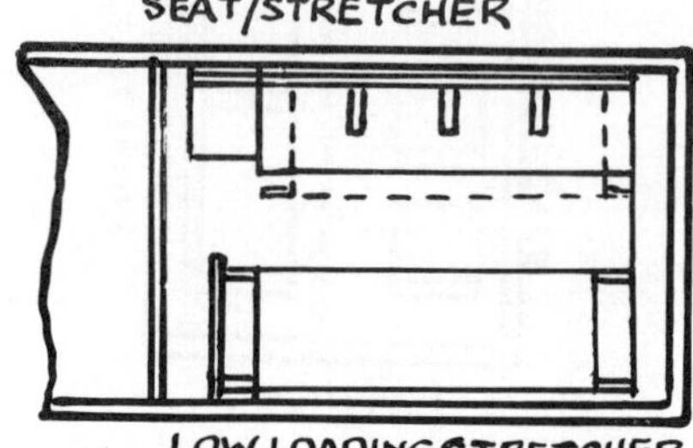

Low loading type stretcher gear on nearside mounted on a locker and incorporating a self-elevating foam bed. Turnover seat/stretcher rack with 3 folding armrests and a light alloy folding stretcher on offside. Attendant's seat fitted in front of turnover stretcher on offside. Accommodation - 4 sitting cases and 1 stretcher case, or 2 stretcher cases.

Body Specification No. 8 (No layout sketches available)

4 standard interior layouts for seats and stretchers -
1. Double berth stretcher racks fitted to both sides giving space for 4 stretcher cases. Backs fold up to expose bench seats. Small tip-up rear-facing seat for attendant. Accommodation - 4 stretcher cases, or 2 stretcher cases and 4 sitting cases, or 8 sitting cases.
2. Double berth stretcher rack fitted to one side and a Multi-Posture model stretcher trolley opposite with backrest and armrests. Attendant's seat as above. Accommodation - 3 stretcher cases, or 2 stretcher cases and 4 sitting cases, or 1 stretcher case and 4 sitting cases, or 8 sitting cases.
3. Two Multi-Posture stretcher trolleys. Attendant's seat as above. Accommodation - 2 stretcher cases, or 1 stretcher case and 4 sitting cases, or 8 sitting cases.
4. One Multi-Posture stretcher trolley one side and turnover seat/stretcher rack opposite, complete with armrests. Attendant's seat as above. Accommodation - 2 stretcher cases, or 1 stretcher case and 4 sitting cases, or 8 sitting cases.
Note: other alternative interior layouts available at customer's request.

Body Specification No. 9

3 standard interior layouts for seats and stretchers -

DOUBLE BERTH STRETCHER

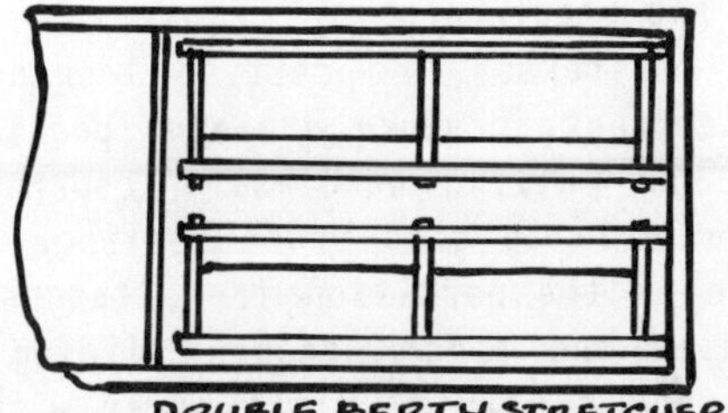

LAYOUT 1

1. Double berth stretcher rack on both sides, giving capacity of 4 stretcher patients. Backs fold up to expose bench type seats. Small rearward facing seat for attendant. Accommodation - 4 stretcher cases, or 2 stretcher cases and 4 sitting cases, or 8 sitting cases.

2. Double berth stretcher rack on one side with stretcher trolley on the other, complete with mattress, backrest and armrests. Seat for attendant as 1. 2 light folding stretchers, 1 pole & canvas type stretcher with spreaders. Accommodation - 3 stretcher cases, or 1 stretcher case and 4 sitting cases, or 8 sitting cases.

3. 2 stretcher trolleys, with mattresses, backrests and armrests. Attendant's seat as 1. 2 pole & canvas type stretchers with spreaders. Accommodation - 2 stretcher cases, or 1 stretcher case and 4 sitting cases, or 8 sitting cases.

Body Specification No. 10
3 standard interior layouts for seats and stretchers -

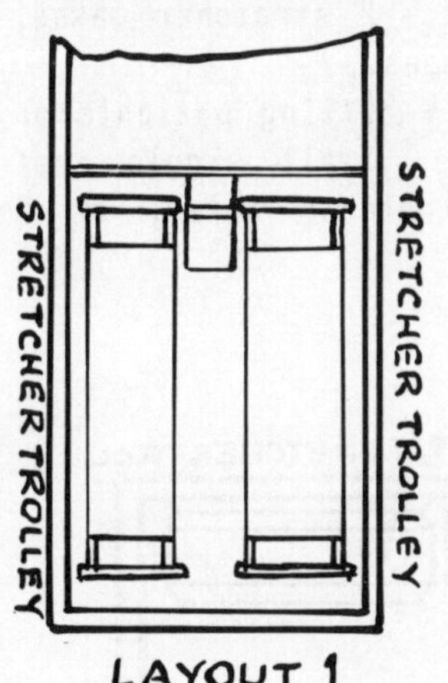

LAYOUT 1

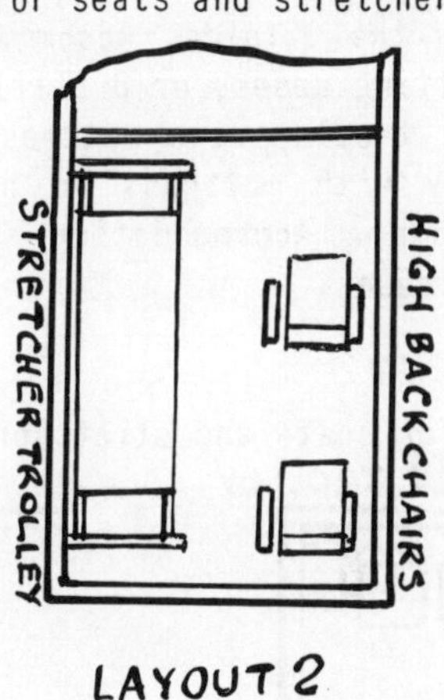

LAYOUT 2

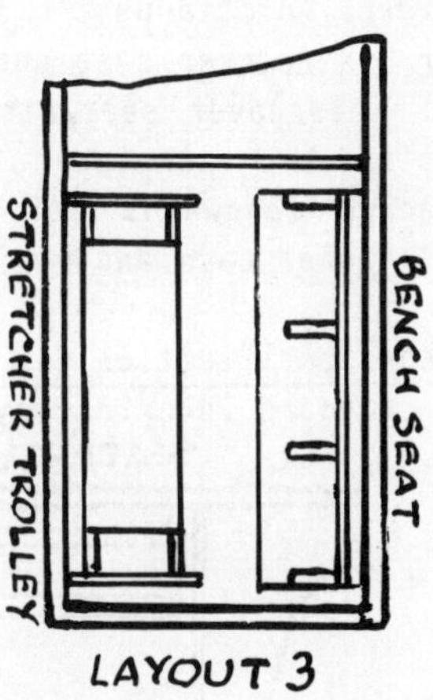

LAYOUT 3

1. 2 stretcher trolleys with mattresses on both sides. Small rearwards facing seat for attendant. Accommodation - 2 stretcher cases.

2. A stretcher trolley with mattress on nearside and 2 high back chairs with armrests on offside. Accommodation - 1 stretcher case and 2 sitting cases.

3. A stretcher trolley with mattress on nearside and a bench seat with backrest and 4 armrests on offside. Accommodation - 1 stretcher case and 3 sitting cases.

Body Specification No. 11 (No layout sketch available.)
A standard interior layout for seats and stretchers.
2 stretcher trolleys, complete with mattresses, 2 position locking devices. Trolleys provide adjustment in the backrest, posture draining position, telescopic handles, folding side rails and pulling handles. A backrest with 4 folding armrests fitted on right hand side to give bench seating. 2 rearward facing tip-up seats on the rear face of the partition for attendants, and a storage locker with adjustable shelves and clear perspex sliding doors. 2 canvas stretchers with spreader bars and a pair of light poles with stowage. Accommodation - 2 stretcher cases, or 1 stretcher case and 3 sitting cases.

Body Specification No. 12
2 standard interior layouts for seats and stretchers -

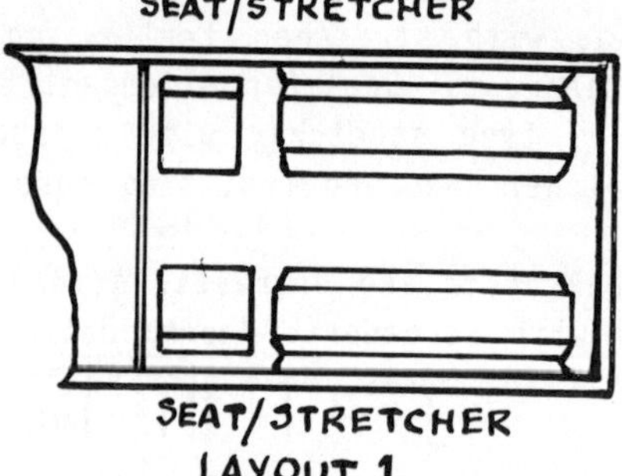

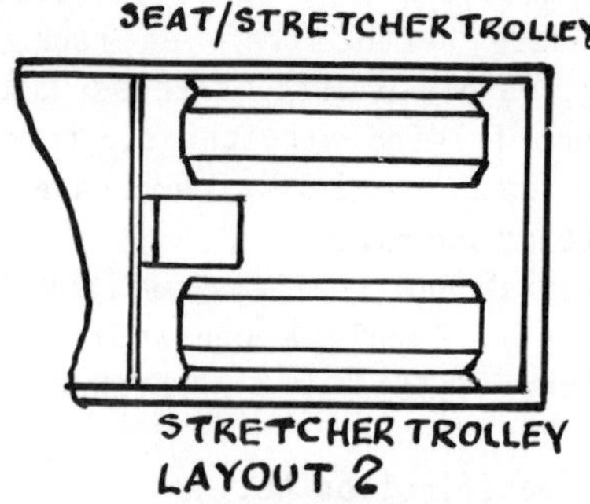

SEAT/STRETCHER
LAYOUT 1
    STRETCHER TROLLEY
LAYOUT 2

1. A turnover seat/stretcher rack with mattress, backrest and armrests on both sides. An attendant's seat on the offside. Accommodation - 2 stretcher cases, or 1 stretcher case and 4 sitting cases, or 8 sitting casses.
2. A turnover seat/stretcher trolley with mattress for 4 sitting patients on offside. A stretcher trolley with mattress on nearside. Small single seat facing rearwards for attendant. Accommodation - 2 stretcher cases, or 1 stretcher case and 4 sitting cases.

Body Specification No. 13
2 standard interior layouts for seats and stretchers -

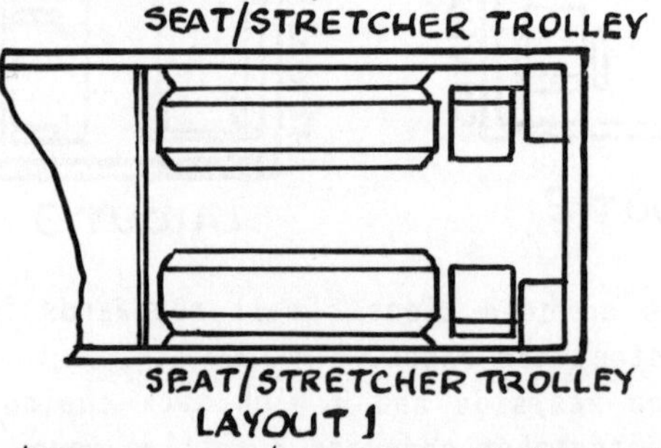

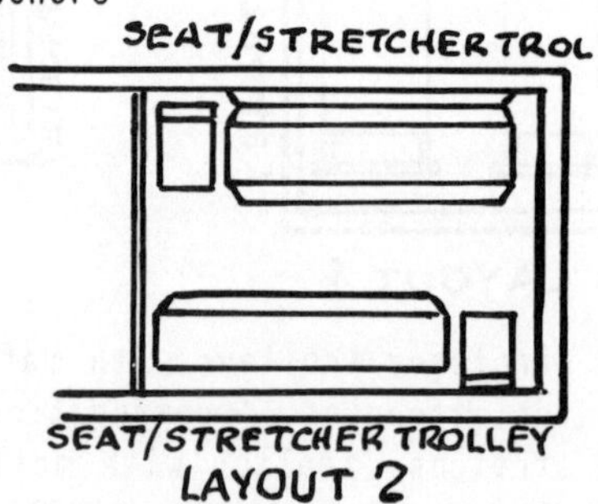

SEAT/STRETCHER TROLLEY
LAYOUT 1
    SEAT/STRETCHER TROLLEY
LAYOUT 2

1. A turnover seat/stretcher trolley with mattress, backrest and armrests to take 4 sitting patients on both sides. Small attendant's seat on both sides to rear of stretcher trolleys. Accommodation - 2 stretcher cases, or 1 stretcher case and 4 sitting cases, or 8 sitting cases.
2. As above, but with the attendant's seat on the offside in front of the stretcher trolley. Accommodation - as above.

SECTION TWO

The following are taken from well-known coachbuilders to show typical contruction of welfare vehicle bodies currently made.

Welfare Body Specification No. 1

This body is based on the Bedford 'CF' range chassis cowl version. 2 wheelbases are available, short at 3.2 metres (126 inches) and long at 3.56 metres (140 inches).

4 standard layouts for seats and invalid wheelchairs -

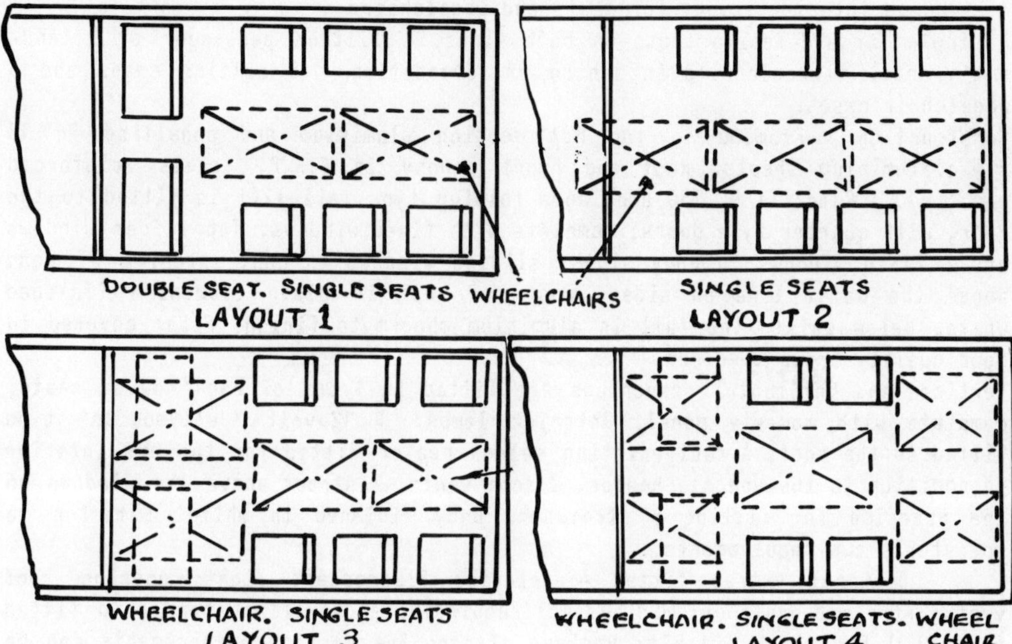

1. A double seat and 3 single seats forward-facing on both side. Two wheelchairs facing forward in the centre. Accommodation - 10 sitting cases and 2 wheelchair cases.

2. 4 single seats facing forward on both sides. 3 wheelchairs facing forward in the centre. Accommodation - 8 sitting cases and 3 wheelchair cases.

3. A wheelchair and 3 forward-facing single seats on both sides. 2 wheelchairs facing forward in the centre. Accommodation - 6 sitting cases and 4 wheelchair cases.

4. A wheelchair facing forward, 2 single forward-facing seats and a wheelchair at the rear on both sides. A wheelchair in the centre. Accommodation - 4 sitting cases and 4 wheelchair cases.

Note: The two latter layouts are based on the first layout by the removal of the double seats and the last 2 single seats as necessary. In the basic layout 1, the first 4 single seats are fixed, while the double and the last 2 single seats are removable.

Construction - Framing and panelling in aluminium for strength, corrosion resistance and lightweight structure. Interior is lined and heated. Lighting is provided. Ventilation is by roof ventilator and hit and miss type interior

grille panel.
Equipment - Tail lifts as requested.
Finish - To the operator's requirements.

Welfare Body Speficiation No. 2

This body is based on the Bedford 'CF' model chassis cowl version. The short wheelbase is used at 3.2 metres (126 inches). Designed to achieve accessibility to load space by wide sliding doors of the cab.
No layout sketch available.
A standard interior layout for seats and wheelchairs -
4 single forward-facing seats on both sides. A tilting passenger or attendant's seat. 3 wheelchairs in centre. Accommodation - 8 sitting cases and 3 wheelchair cases.
Construction - Framing in top hat section aluminium and panelling in 18 s.w.g.aluminium sheets. Roof and front canopy in G.R.P. (glass reinforced plastic). A Ratcliff RF 250 ambulance folding type tail lift is fitted to the rear, with quarter type doors, complete with fixed windows. Top slider windows and 2 fixed windows in body sides, sliding windows in cab. Interior of body above the waist line on sides, roof and rear in plain aluminium finished white. Below waist line rail in aluminium checkmate finish. Floor covered in good quality brown linoleum.
Vertical and horizontal stanchions are fitted in front of each row of seats, complete with modesty panel. Interior lamps: 3 12-volt 'Jellymoulds' type fitted in the roof. A recirculating saloon heater fitted for the bus interior in addition to the vehicle heater. 2 roof vents. 2 straps above the windows on the nearside for fitting a stretcher. Body finished in white. Exterior to operator's own requirements.
          Optional extras fitted - interior fluorescent light; opening roof vents; fire extinguisher; Minibus Act requirements; auxiliary hand pump fitted to tail lift; first aid kit; various alternative seating arrangements can be negotiated and paint schemes, including sign writing to suit operators.

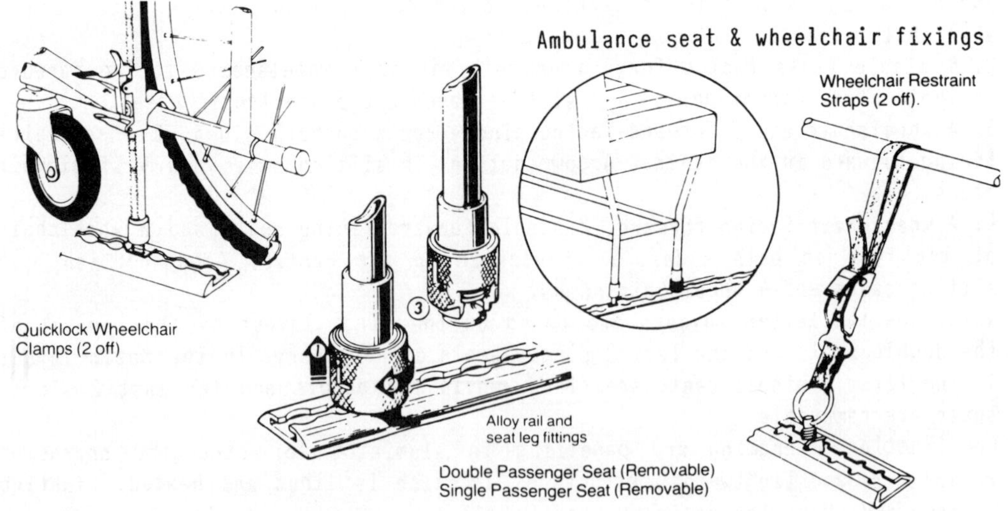

Welfare Body Specification No. 3

This bus body is based on the Bedford 'CF30' chassis cowl version, 3.2 metre (126 inches) wheelbase with 2.3 litre petrol engine, incorporating a flat floor for ease of wheelchair accommodation.

4 standard layouts similar to those in Specification No. 1.

Construction - Zinc coated steel sections and steel panelling. Sliding cab doors. Twin hinged rear doors. Electro hydraulically operated tail lift. Permanent roof ventilation. Top sliding windows in centre of body sides. Sliding cab door windows. Cab and passenger compartment heaters. Anchor points to secure wheelchairs.

Welfare Body Specification No. 4

Based on the Ford 'A' Series models AO609 chassis windshield version with the 3.5 litre diesel engine, and the AO610 chassis windshield version with the 3.0 litre petrol engine.

4 standard interior layouts for seats and wheelchairs -

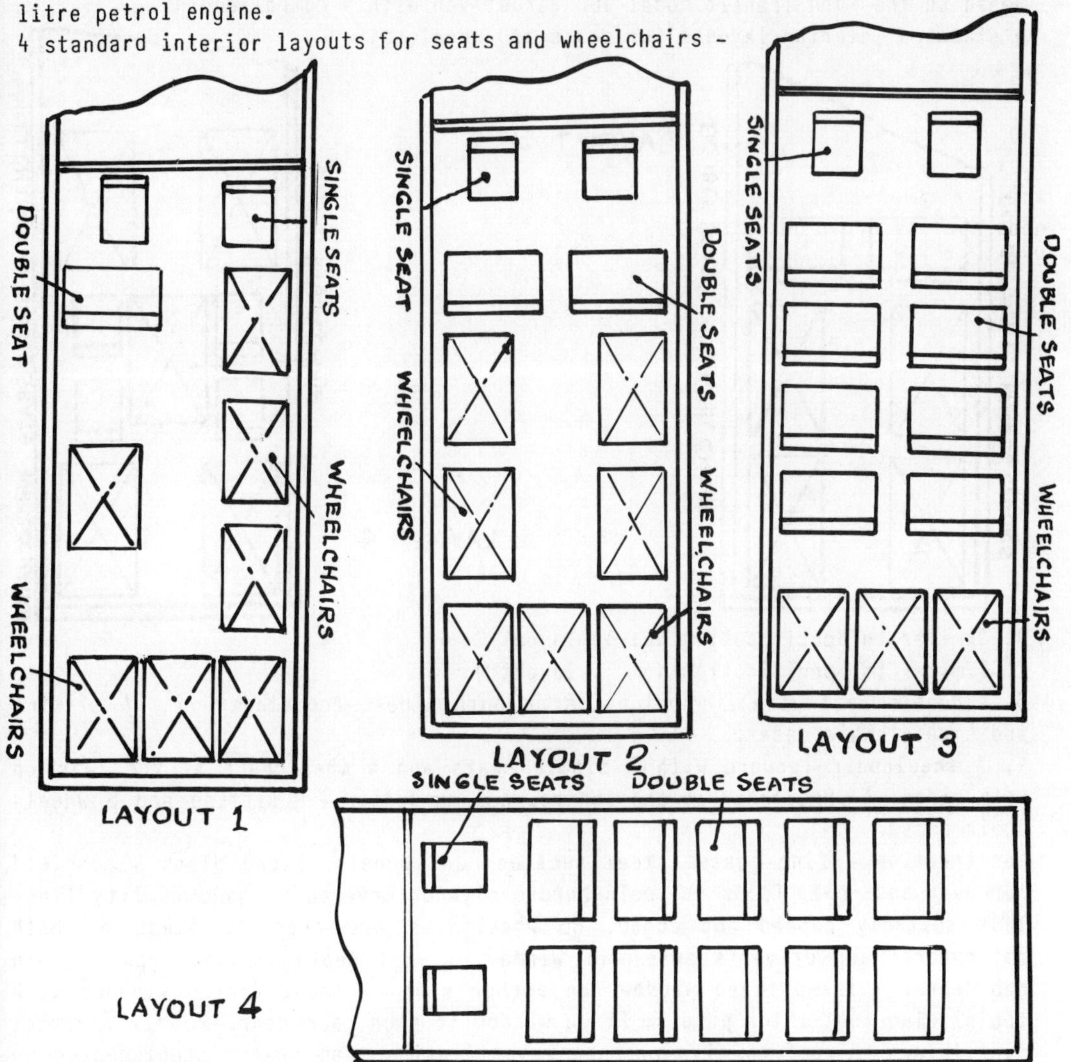

1. A removable double seat, a removable single seat at front, a wheelchair midway at nearside. 3 wheelchairs on offside. 3 wheelchairs across the rear. Accommodation - 4 sitting cases and 7 wheelchair cases.
2. A double seat and 2 wheelchairs, an attendant's seat at the front on both sides. 3 wheelchairs across the rear. Accommodation - 4 sitting and 7 wheelchair cases.
3. 4 double seats on both sides. 3 wheelchairs across rear. Accommodation - 16 sitting and 3 wheelchair cases.
4. 5 double seats on both sides. Accommodation - 20 sitting cases.
Construction and Finish - similar to Specification No. 3.
Note: in all these layouts there are 2 attendants' seats at the front.

Welfare Body Specification No. 5

Based on the Ford Transit model 160 Parcel Van with a petrol engine.
4 standard interior layouts for seats and wheelchairs -

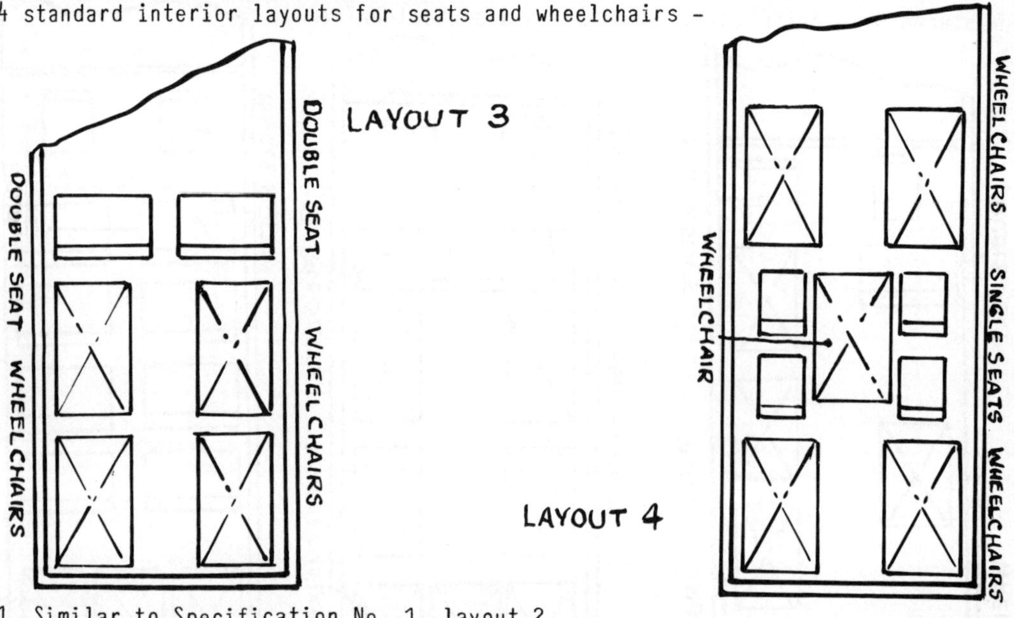

1. Similar to Specification No. 1, layout 2.
2. Similar to Specification No. 1, layout 1.
3. A double seat with 2 wheelchairs on both sides. Accommodation - 4 sitting and 4 wheelchair cases.
4. A wheelchair forward with 2 single seats and a wheelchair at the rear on both sides. A wheelchair in the centre. Accommodation - 4 sitting and 5 wheelchair cases.
Construction - Zinc coated steel sections and panels. Fibre glass windshield surround and roof. Floor in resin bonded plywood covered in good quality linoleum suitably capped and edged. No wheelboxes are present. Steps at both passengers' and driver's entrance. Window of full depth sliding type to both cab doors. 3 large fixed windows on either side of body. Centre windows with top sliding ventilator panels. Fixed window to each rear door. 2 inlet/extract ventilators to roof to give permanent ventilation. Cab heater supplemented by

a hot water recirculator heater for the ambulance compartment. 3 'Jellymould' tungsten lamps are fitted to the interior roof lining panels and a loading lamp is fitted to illuminate the tail lift entrance. There are inertia reel seat belts for the driver and the attendant, wheelchair restaints are also provided. Twin column tail lift 250 kg (551½ lb). Folding stretcher and stowage. Simulated wood grain finish laminated between floor and windows. Exterior mirrors L.H. and R.H. fitted to front pillars. Aeon assistor springs in the suspension. Body exterior on single colour as required, interior in white, roof panels white impregnated G.R.P., underside of body black preservative paint. Seating shark grey. Floor covering red and seat frames in matt black.

<u>Welfare BodySpecificationNo. 6</u>
Based on the Dodge model D955.
6 standard interior layouts for seats and wheelchairs –
1. Similar to Specification No. 4, layout 1.

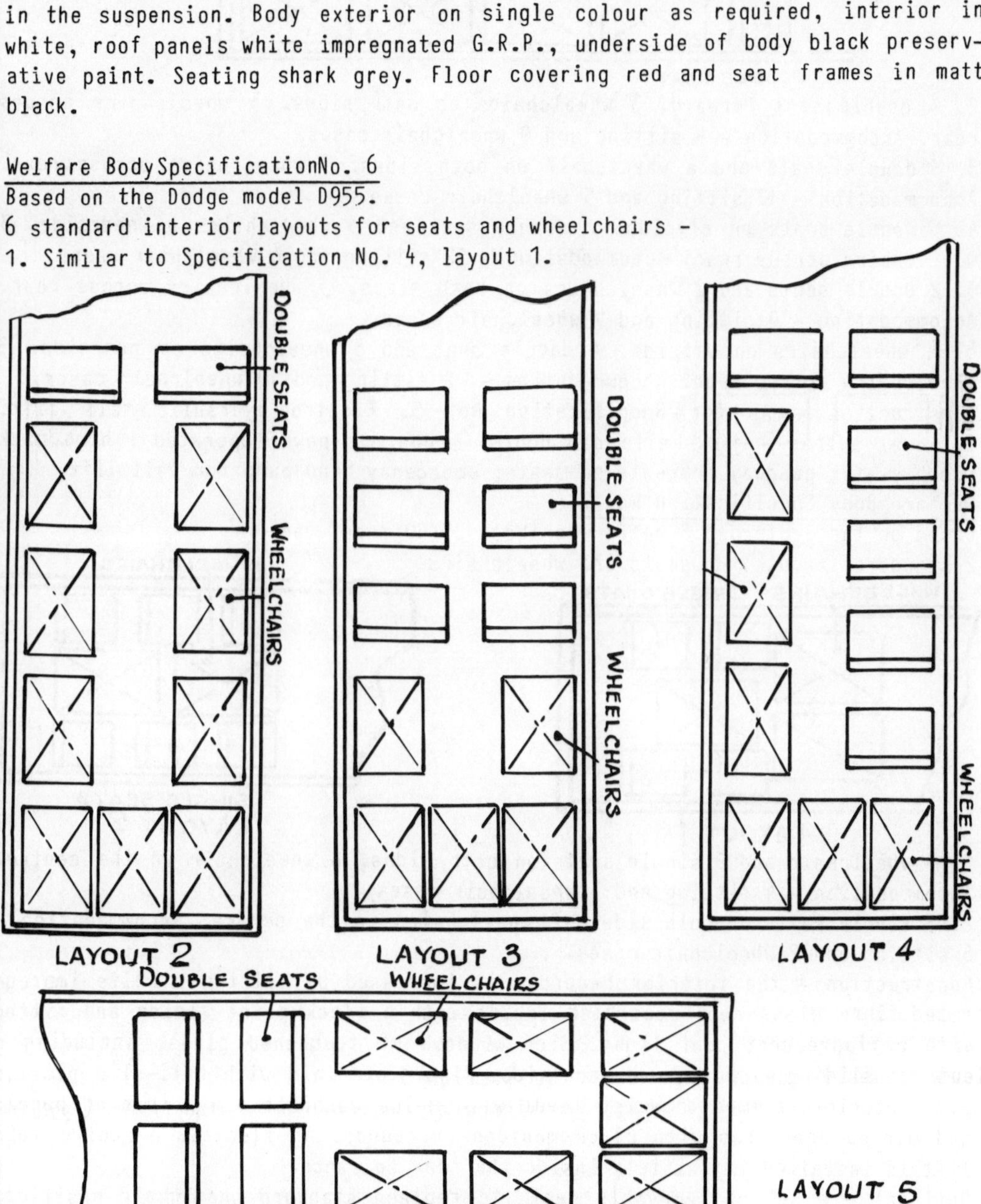

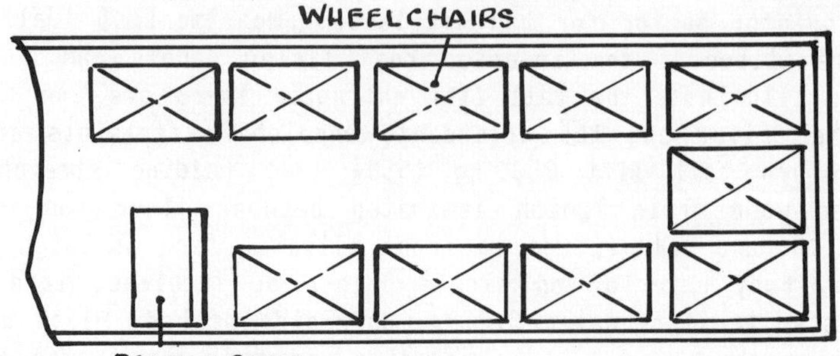

2. A double seat forward, 3 wheelchairs on both sides. 3 wheelchairs across rear. Accommodation - 4 sitting and 9 wheelchair cases.

3. 3 double seats and a wheelchair on both sides. 3 wheelchairs across rear. Accommodation - 12 sitting and 5 wheelchair cases.

4. 5 double seats on offside. A double seat and 3 wheelchairs on nearside. 3 wheelchairs across rear. Accommodation - 12 sitting and 6 wheelchair cases.

5. 2 double seats and 2 wheelchairs on both sides. 3 wheelchairs across rear. Accommodation - 8 sitting and 7 wheelchair cases.

6. 4 wheelchairs on offside. A double seat and 3 wheelchairs on nearside. 3 wheelchairs across rear. Accommodation - 2 sitting and 10 wheelchair cases.

Construction - As for Specification No. 5. Electro hydraulic tail lift. Optional extras - jack-knife cab doors (manual or power operated); high back coach seats; gangway armrests on seats; emergency hand pump for tail lift.

Welfare Body Specification No. 7

Based on the Bedford 3.2 metre wheelbase CF280 model van.

2 standard layouts for seats and wheelchairs

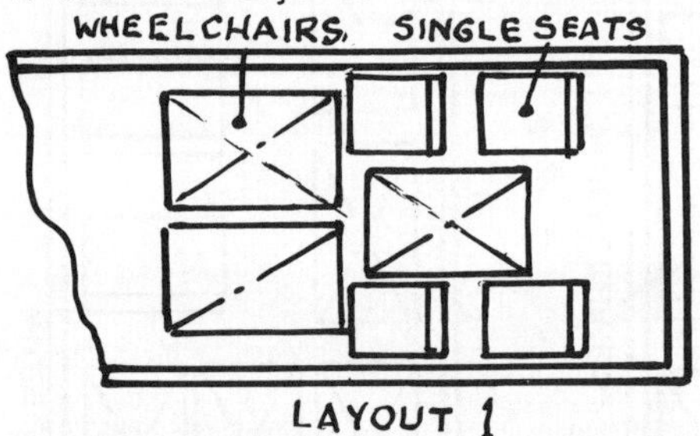

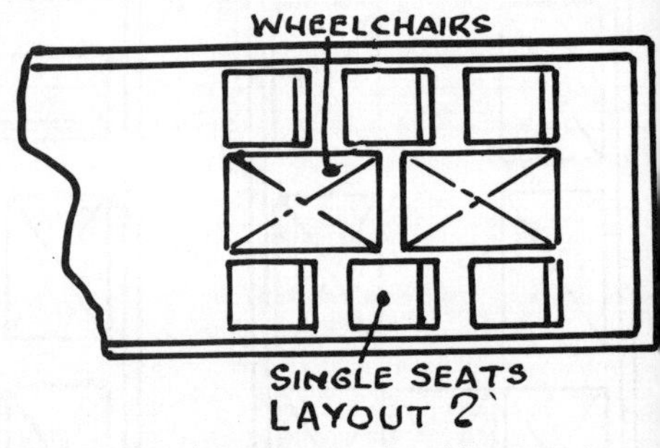

1. A wheelchair and 2 single seats on both sides. A wheelchair in the centre. Accommodation - 4 sitting and 3 wheelchair cases.

2. 3 single seats on both sides. 2 wheelchairs in the centre. Accommodation - 6 sitting and 2 wheelchair cases.

Construction - the interior headroom is increased by fitting a white impregnated fibre glass roof decorated inside with a fleck paint finish and fitted with a fluorescent roof light. Side windows of toughened glass, including a pair of sliding windows, one each side. Floors overlaid with anti-slip plastic ply. Interior trimmed to waist level with beige washable vinyl covered panels and window apertures with black moulded surrounds. An electric hyraulic tail lift is installed immediately inside the rear entrance.

Optional - a set of removable seats to replace standard wheelchair positions (increasing the accommodation for sitting cases), small windows in the sides of the extended roof.

A similar specification is available for the Ford Transit models.

Welfare Body Specification No. 8
Based on several vehicles including Bedford 'CF', Leyland Sherpa, and Ford Transit van and parcel van.

2 standard interior layouts for the seats and wheelchairs.

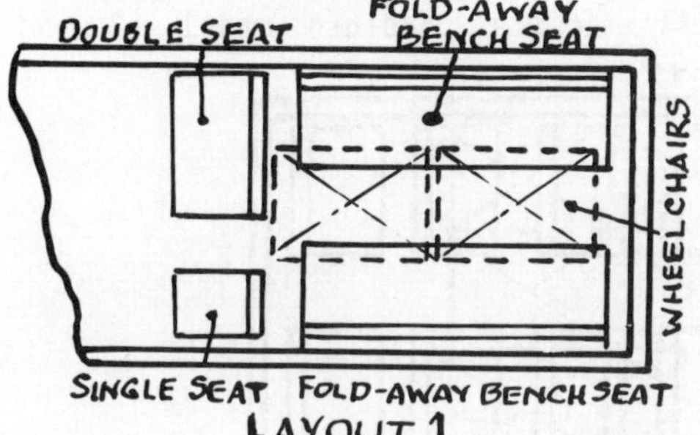

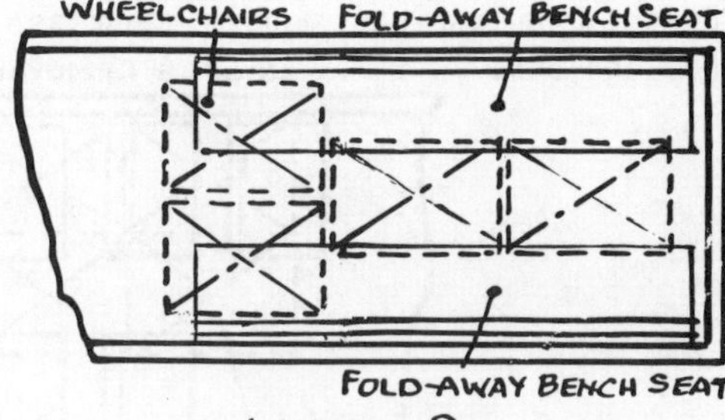

1. Double seat and foldaway bench seat on offside. Single seat and foldaway bench seat on nearside. 2 wheelchairs can be carried if the bench seats are folded away. Accommodation - 11 sitting cases, or 3 sitting and 2 wheelchair cases.

2. A foldaway bench seat on both sides. 4 wheelchairs can be carried if the seats are folded away. Accommodation - 12 sitting cases, or 4 wheelchairs.

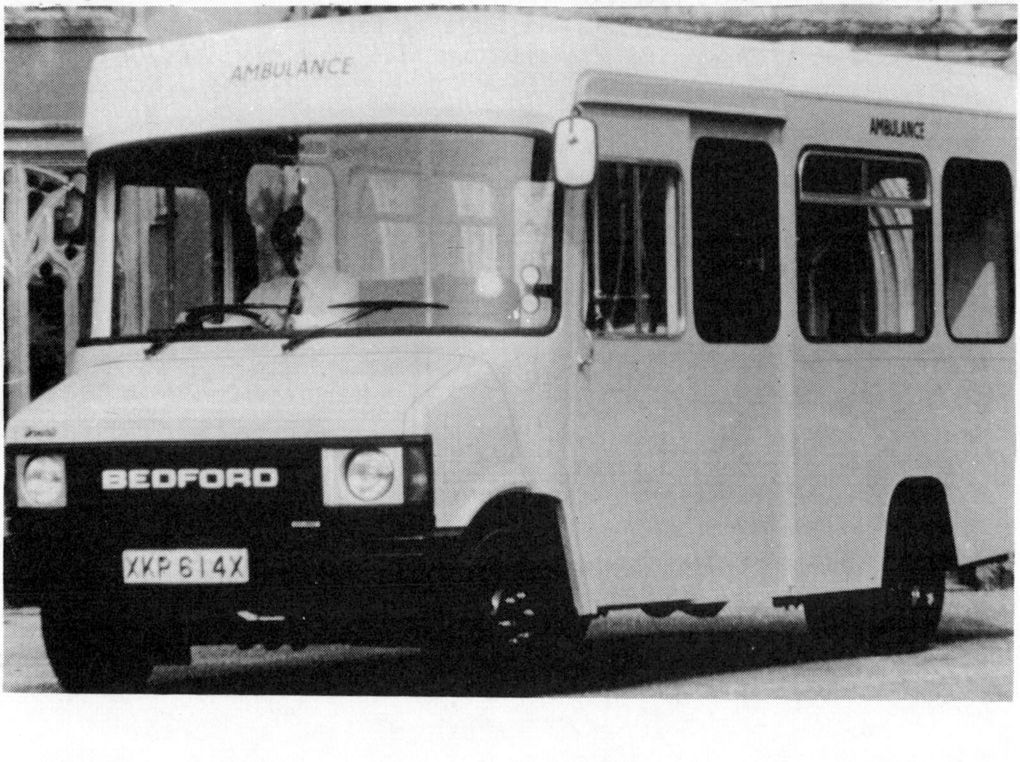

Construction - The conversion feature is the raised roof section with increase in height access doors at the rear. Fold-away electro hydraulically operated tail lift, as well as safety glass side windows. Seats can be tip-up bench type or single, both facing forward and with armrests. With seats folded up, all models have provision for wheelchairs using quick action clamps or a restraint by means of wheel cups with cover plates. Standard fitting included translucent roof panels and recirculating body heaters. There were a range of special options at the operator's request.

Welfare Body Specification No. 9

Based upon various models such as Ford 'A' series, Bedford model SB and Leyland Cub.

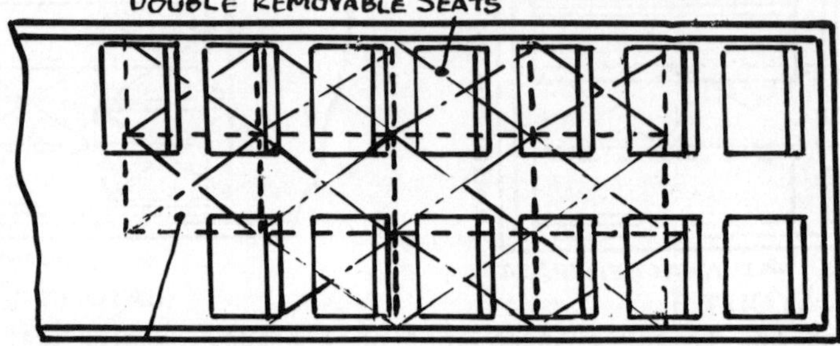

7 double removable seats on offside. 6 double removable seats on nearside. When the seats are removed 14 wheelchairs can be carried. Accommodation - 26 sitting cases, or 14 wheelchairs.
Construction - Aluminium panels on a multiple ring steel body frame. Specially made double seats, fully adjustable and removable to allow wheelchairs to replace them. Front end and rear styling is in G.R.P., with double doors at back enclosing an electro hydraulic tail lift.
Smaller versions of this type are available to suit Ford 'A' series chassis front end, of up to 24 seating accommodation. Also larger versions, with up to 44 seats, based on the Leyland Cub.

Welfare Body Specification No. 10

This is smaller than Specification No. 9, based on the Ford 'A' series.
2 standard interior layouts for seats and wheelchairs-

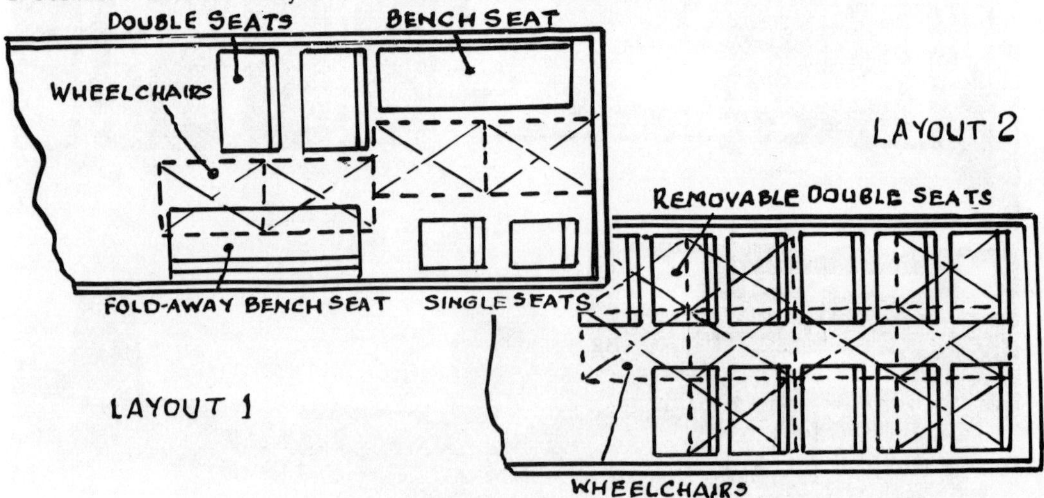

1. 2 double seats and a bench seat on offside. A fold-away type bench seat and
2 single seats on nearside. Accommodation - 12 sitting and 2 wheelchair cases,
or 9 sitting and 4 wheelchair cases.
2. 6 double seats, which are removable, on offside. 5 double seats, also
removable, on nearside. When seats are taken out 9 wheelchairs can be carried.
Accommodation - 22 sitting cases, or 9 wheelchairs.
Welfare Body Specification No. 11

Purpose built to suit the Bedford 'CF' and the Ford Transit front ends,
specially prepared for this type of operation.
2 Standard interior layouts for seats and wheelchairs -

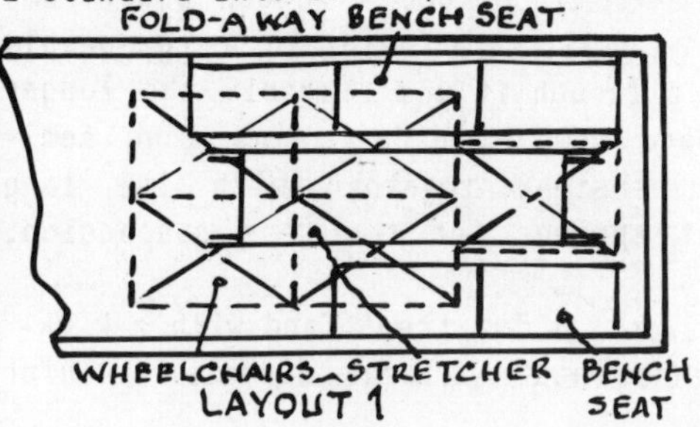

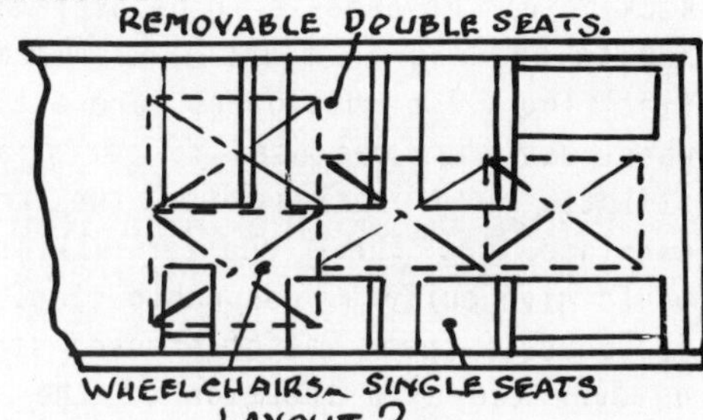

1. 3 double fold-away seats on offside, facing inwards. 2 double fold-away
seats facing inwards on nearside. When seats are folded away 5 wheelchairs can
be carried. Accommodation - 10 sitting cases, or 5 wheelchairs.
2. 3 double seats facing forward and a double seat facing inwards, all removable on offside. An inward facing single seat, 2 forward facing double seats
and an inward facing double seat, all removable, on nearside. When seats are
taken out 4 wheelchairs can be carried. Accommodation - 13 sitting cases, or 5
sitting and 4 wheelchair cases.

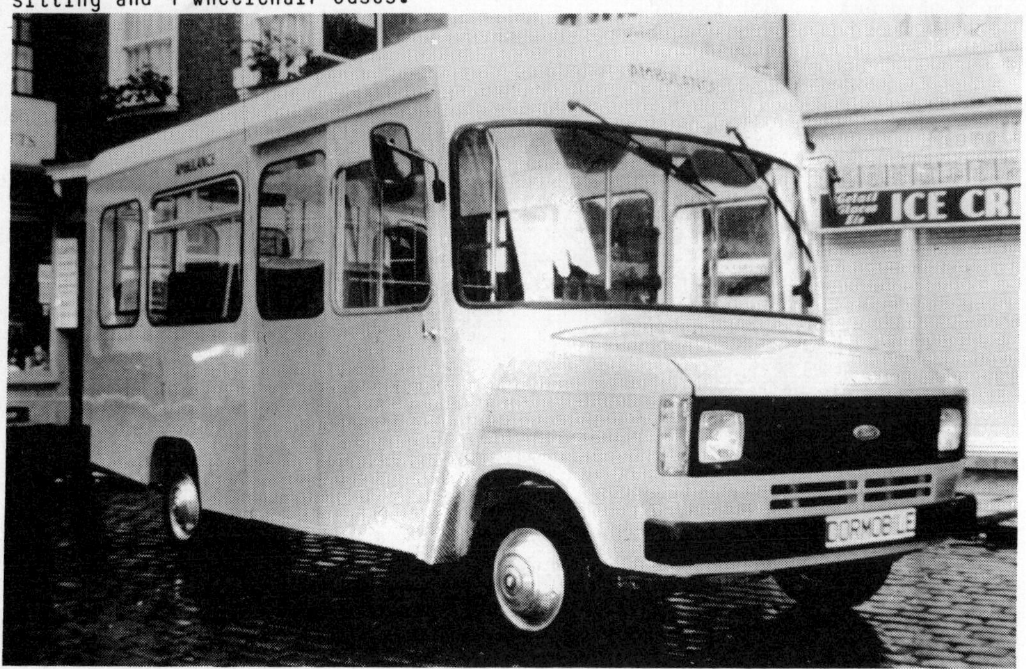

SECTION THREE

These descriptions and brief specifications are for some of the basic vehicles for either conversion of standard vans or chassis versions for the mounting of ambulance or welfare vehicle bodies.

Crossley 20/25 h.p. motor car chassis

The chassis form with the bulk head panel and bonnet of this particular model heavy motor car, formed the basis of a mounted ambulance body. Due to the kick-up of the chassis frame over the rear axle location, a wooden underframe had to be used to mount the ambulance body and try to maintain a reasonably flat floor. Two wheelbases were available, although it was probably the longer wheelbase that was used to carry a standard army stretcher. The long semi-elliptic leaf springs for the front suspension, together with the long carriage type three quarter elliptic leaf springs for the rear suspension, would give quite a reasonable ride.

The chassis frame was of pressed steel, inswept at the front, and with a kick-up over the axle location at the rear, stiffened by large diameter tubular crossmembers.

SPECIFICATION

Engine	Petrol. 4 cylinder, in-line. 4.54 litre
	Rated @ 20/25 h.p. (RAC rating @ 25.6 h.p.)
Wheelbase	Short 3.2 m (126 inch)
	Long 3.43 m (135 inch)
Suspension	Front Semi-elliptic leaf springs
	Rear three quarter elliptic leaf springs
Shock absorbers	Not fitted
Transmission	4 speed, constant mesh. Crash type

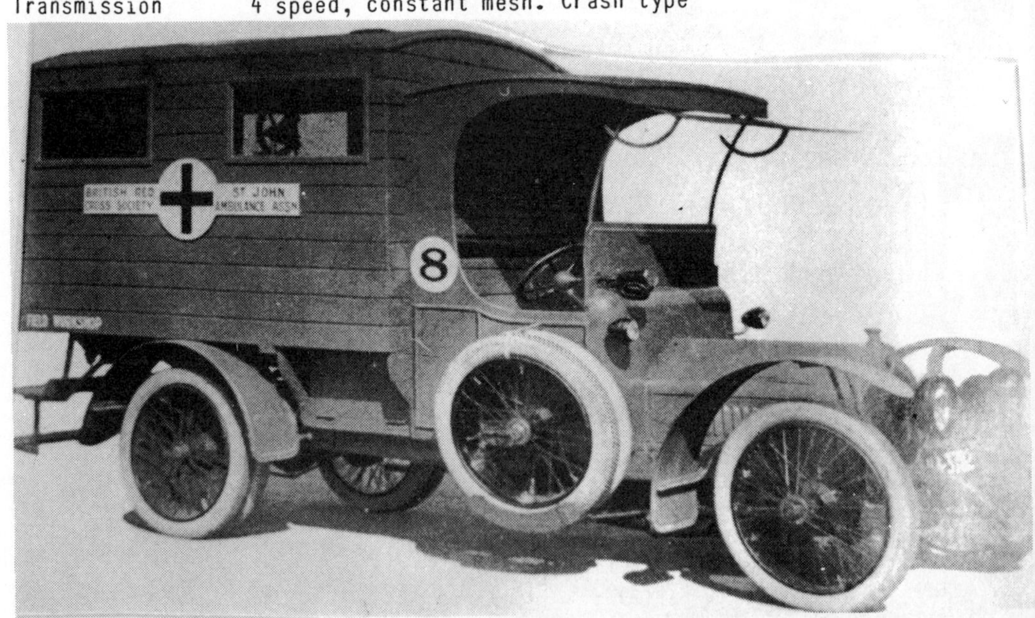

Tyres	880 x 120 Short wheelbase
	895 x 120 Long wheelbase
Dimensions (chassis)	
Overall length	4.52 m (178 inch) Short wheelbase
	4.75 m (187 inch) Long wheelbase
Overall width	1.75 m (69 inches)
Front overhang	0.527 m (20.75 inches) approx.
Rear overhang	0.559 m (22 inches) approx.
Dimensions (with ambulance body)	
	Vary according to body fitted
Weights	
Chassis	Not available
Kerb weight	Vary according to ambulance body

Ford Model 'T'

Used in its chassis front end form with bulk head and bonnet. One wheelbase only. The transverse semi-elliptic leaf springs for the front and rear suspension gave what was termed a 'reasonable ride'. Probably the most used ambulance during the 1914-18 war.

The chassis frame was of pressed steel with the minimum of crossmembers and was fairly flexible.

SPECIFICATION

Engine	Petrol. 4 cylinder in-line. 2.85 litre rated at 20 h.p. @ 1,600 r.p.m.
Wheelbase	2.54 m (100 inches)

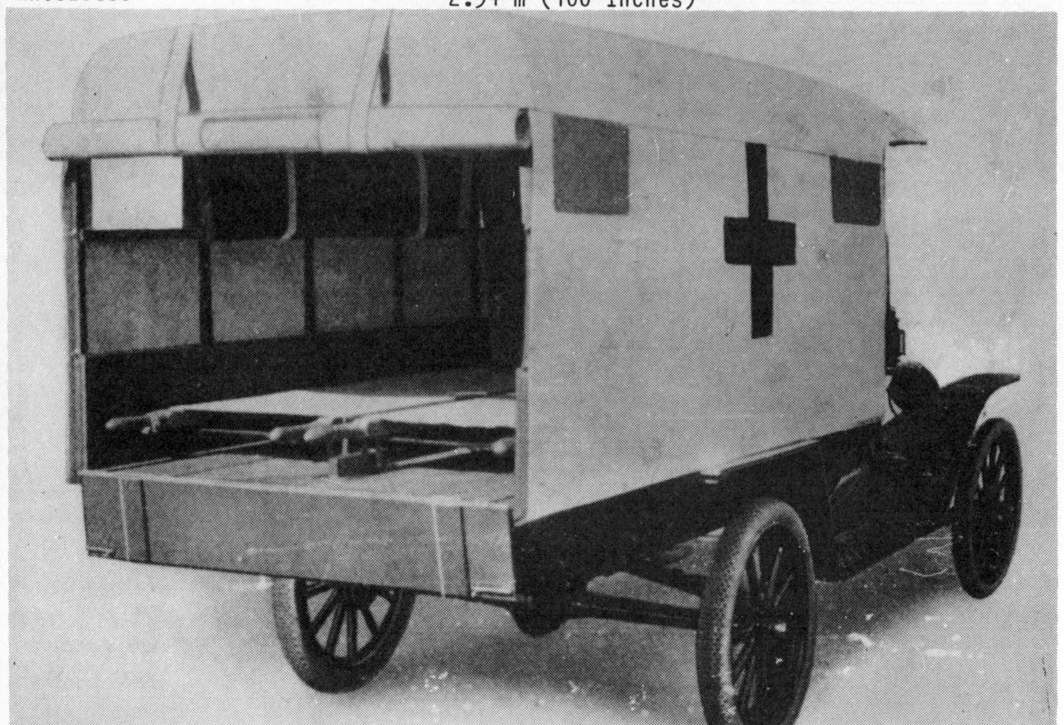

Suspension	Front & rear: transverse semi-elliptic leaf springs
Shock absorbers	Not fitted
Transmission	2 speed. Epicyclic (planetary gears)
Tyres	762mm x 76.2mm (30 x 3 inch) Front
	762mm x 89mm (30 x 3.5 inch) Rear

Dimensions (chassis)

Overall length	4.115 m (162 inches)
	1.371 m (54 inches)
Overall width	Not available
Front overhang	Not available
Rear overhang	2.083 m (82 inches)

Weights

Chassis	585 Kg (1288 lb)
Kerb weight	1175 Kg (2588 lb)

Dennis Brothers (now Hestair Dennis)

This ambulance was specially designed and built in 1915 by Dennis as the most perfect ambulance of its day. One wheelbase only. With the semi-elliptic leaf spring for the front suspension and the cantilever type long semi-elliptic leaf springs for the rear suspension a good comfortable ride was expected. Normal control type. With ladder chassis frame narrowing at the front to give the good front wheel lock for minimum turning circle and with the wide frame towards the rear to give the maximum width of ambulance compartment.

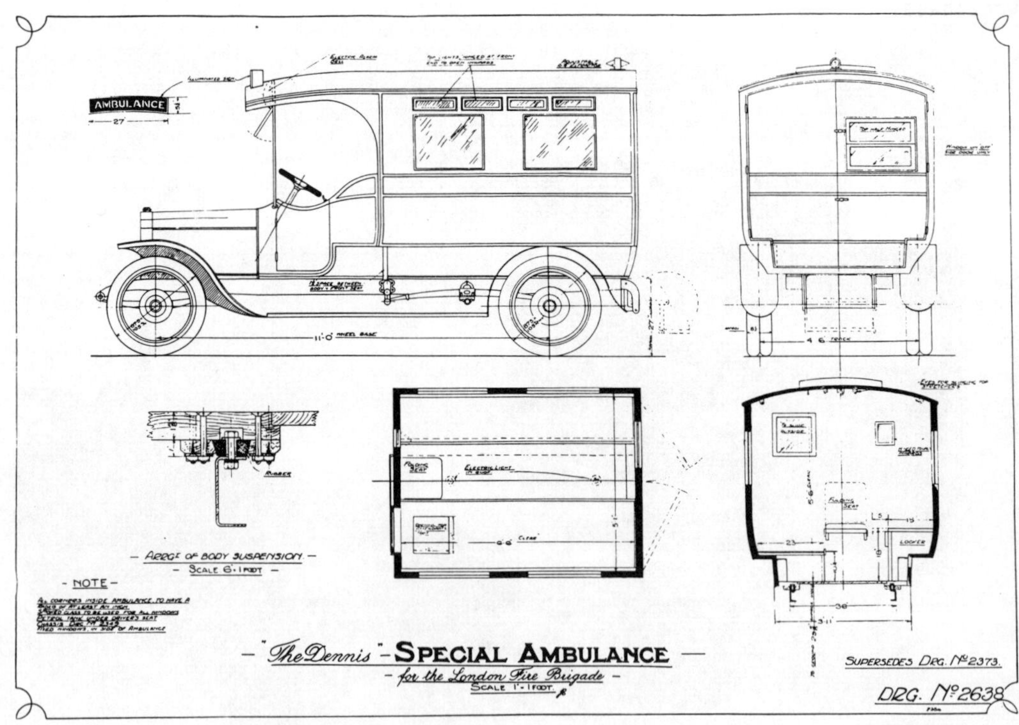

SPECIFICATION
Engine   Petrol. 4 cylinder, in-line. 4.08 litre
                                Develops 28 h.p. @ 1,000 r.p.m.
Wheelbase   3.35 m (132 inches)
                                Front semi-elliptic leaf springs
Suspension   Rear cantilever type semi-elliptic leaf springs
Shock absorbers   Not fitted
Transmission   4 speed Constant mesh Crash type
Tyres   895 x 135mm (35.24 x 5.31 inch) 2 non-
                                skid type fitted. All with detachable rims.

Dimensions (chassis)
      Overall length   4.77 m (188 inches)

      Overall width   1.75 m (69 inches)
      Front overhang   0.61 m (24 inches)
      Rear overhang   0.812 m (32 inches)
Dimensions (with ambulance body) 2.59 m (102 inches)
Weights
      Chassis   1143 Kg (2529 lb)
      Kerb weight   3124 Kg (6880 lb)

Dennis Brothers (Hestair Dennis)

Model A.V. 1954 to 56. In production till late 1960s.
Chassis with front end engine cover and front floor. Special features, Gegoire
patent suspension system on rear axle, which provided a coil spring mounted in
association with the normal semi-elliptic leaf spring. Upward movement of the
rear axle, or conversely, downward movement of the body, puts the coil springs
in tension which increases as the magnitude of the oscillations. The effect of
this combination of springs was to give the system a variable rate to cushion
shock progressively. Violence of movement in either direction was countered by
the presence of hydraulic shock absorbers. The engine unit and the gearbox
were carried on a four point flexible mounting system.
SPECIFICATION
Engine   Petrol. 4 cylinder, in-line. 2.844 litre
                                78 b.h.p. 3,750 r.p.m. (Rolls Royce engine B40)
                                (appeared in 1956 as optional unit to diesel engine)
                                Diesel. 4 cylinder, in-line. 3.16 litre
                                60 b.h.p. @ 3,000 r.p.m. (Perkins P4)
Wheelbase   2.667 m (105 inches)
Suspension   Front Semi-elliptic leaf springs
                                Rear Coil springs & semi-elliptic leaf springs
Shock absorbers   Double acting, hydraulic. Telescopic
                                type on front. Lever arm type rear.
Transmission   4 speed, synchromesh. Manual.
Tyres   7.00 x 16 - 8 ply rating
Dimensions (chassis)
      Overall length   4.52 m (178 inches)
      Overall width   1.99 m (78.5 inches)
      Front overhang   1.079 m (42.5 inches)

Rear overhang	0.774 m (30.5 inches)

Dimensions (with ambulance body)

Vary with ambulance body fitted

Weights

Chassis	1193 Kg (2632 lb)
Kerb weight	2416 Kg (5328 lb)

Transport Vehicles (Daimler) Ltd. [Jaguar Cars]

Produced in the early 50s, the Daimler ambulance was one of the more popular vehicles of its kind. Specially designed in collaboration with the medical and municipal authorities. One wheelbase only. With coil springs and a torsional stabiliser type front suspension and long semi-elliptic leaf springs for the rear gave a very comfortable ride and good handling qualities. The drive was through a fluid flywheel coupling to a pre-selector gearbox. The rear axle drive was offset to the nearside to help in maintaining a low flat floor and rear entrance.

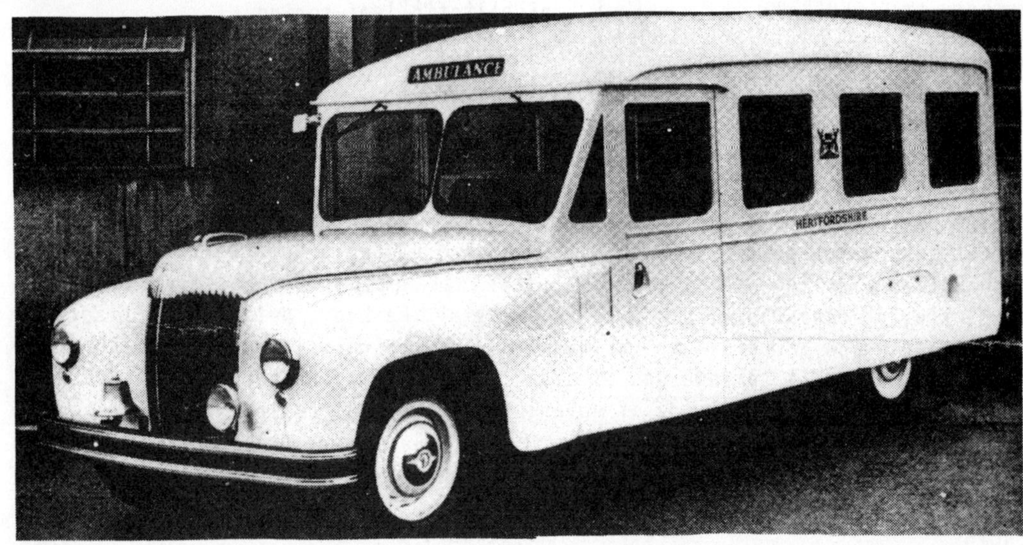

SPECIFICATION

Engine	Petrol. 4 cylinder, in-line. 4.09 litre.
	110 b.h.p. @ 3,600 r.p.m.
Wheelbase	3.81 m (150 inches)
	Front: Coil springs with torsional stabiliser
Suspension	Rear: Semi-elliptic springs
Shock absorbers	Double acting hydraulic. Lever arm type f & r
Transmission	4 speed epicyclic pre-selector gearbox with fluid flywheel coupling
Tyres	8.00 x 17 Single rear equipment

Dimensions (with ambulance body)

Overall length	5.74 m (226 inches)
Overall width	1.98 m (78 inches)
Front overhang	Not available
Rear overhang	Not available

| | Overall height | 2.311 m (91 inches) |

Weights
| | Chassis | 2019 Kg (4452 lb) |
| | Kerb weight | 3251 Kg (7168 lb) |

Morris Commercial (British Leyland)

1963 conversion of the basic Morris van, supplied with driver's and passengers' seats, to ambulance model 'J4-M10'. Forward control with access to engine, etc., via an engine cover inside driver's compartment.

SPECIFICATION

Engine	Petrol 4 cylinder, in-line. 1.622 litre
	B.H.P. not available.
	Diesel 4 cylinder, in-line. 1,459 litre
	40 B.H.P. @ 4,000 r.p.m.
Wheelbase	2.286 m (90 inches)
	Front Independent coil spring
Suspension	Rear Semi-elliptic leaf spring
Shock absorbers	Double acting, hydraulic. Lever arm type
Transmission	4 speed synchromesh
Tyres	6.40 x 14.Single rear equipment

Dimensions (With Wadham Stringer body)
	Overall length	4.103 m (158 inches)
	Overall width	1.765 m (69.5 inches)
	Front overhang	Not available
	Rear overhang	Not available

Weights
| | Chassis | Not available |
| | Kerb weight | 2059 Kg (4540 lb) |

'J2-M16'. 1965

1965 conversion of the basic Morris van, supplied with hinged cab and rear doors, driver's and passengers' seats. With or without side loading doors. Forward control with access to the engine, etc., via an engine cover inside driver's compartment.

SPECIFICATION

Engine	Petrol. 4 cylinder, in-line. 1.498 litre
	42.8 b.h.p. @ 4,000 r.p.m.
	Diesel 4 cylinder, in-line. 1.498 litre
	40 b.h.p. @ 4,000 r.p.m.
Wheelbase	2.286 m (90 inches)
	Front Independent coil spring
Suspension	Rear Semi-elliptic leaf springs
Shock absorbers	Double acting, hydraulic
Transmission	4 speed synchromesh
Tyres	6.50 x 15 6 ply rating tubeless. Single rear equipment
	6.75 x 15 optional

Dimensions (with Wadham Stringer body)
| | Overall length | 4.013 m (158 inches) |

Overall width	1.765 (69.5 inches)
Front overhang	Not available
Rear overhang	Not available

Weights

Chassis	Not available
Kerb weight	Not available

'J2-M16'. 1966

1966 chassis front end and windshield version of the Morris van. Supplied to body builder with loose hinged cab doors, driver's and passengers' seats and fitted floor. Forward control with access to the engine, etc., by an engine cover in the driver's compartment.

As for the 'J2-M16' 1965 , except for
Overall height   2.375 m (93.5 inches)

Austin Motor Company (Austin Rover)

The standard Austin 3 litre car, saloon, 1970, with 6 cylinder engine. Converted into an ambulance for duties with either small or private hospitals.

SPECIFICATION

Engine	Petrol. 6 cylinder, in-line. 2.912 litre. B.H.P. not available.
Wheelbase	2.947 m (116 inches)
Suspension	Front Independent wishbone Hydrolastic unit Rear Independent trailing arm. Hydrolastic unit
Shock absorbers	Armstrong levelling device
Transmission	4 speed synchromesh plus overdrive Automatic transmission (Borg Warner) optional

Dimensions (With Wadham Stringer body)

Overall length	4.725 m (186 inches)
Overall width	1.702 m (67 inches)
Front overhang	Not available
Rear overhang	Not available
Overall height	1.626 m (64 inches)

Weights

Chassis	Not available
Kerb weight	1270 Kg (2800 lb)

British Motor Corporation (BMC)

Special model 250JU. Chassis cab version. With petrol or diesel engine. One wheelbase. Forward control. Underfloor engine.

SPECIFICATION

Engine	Petrol 4 cylinder, in-line. 1.622 litre. B.h.p. not available Diesel 4 cylinder, in-line 1,489 litre 40.0 b.h.p. @ 4,000 r.p.m.
Wheelbase	2.947 m (116 inches)
Suspension	Front & rear Semi-elliptic leaf springs
Shock absorbers	Double acting, hydraulic, telescopic f & r
Transmission	4 speed synchromesh
Tyres	7.00 x 16 6 ply rating. Single tyre equipment

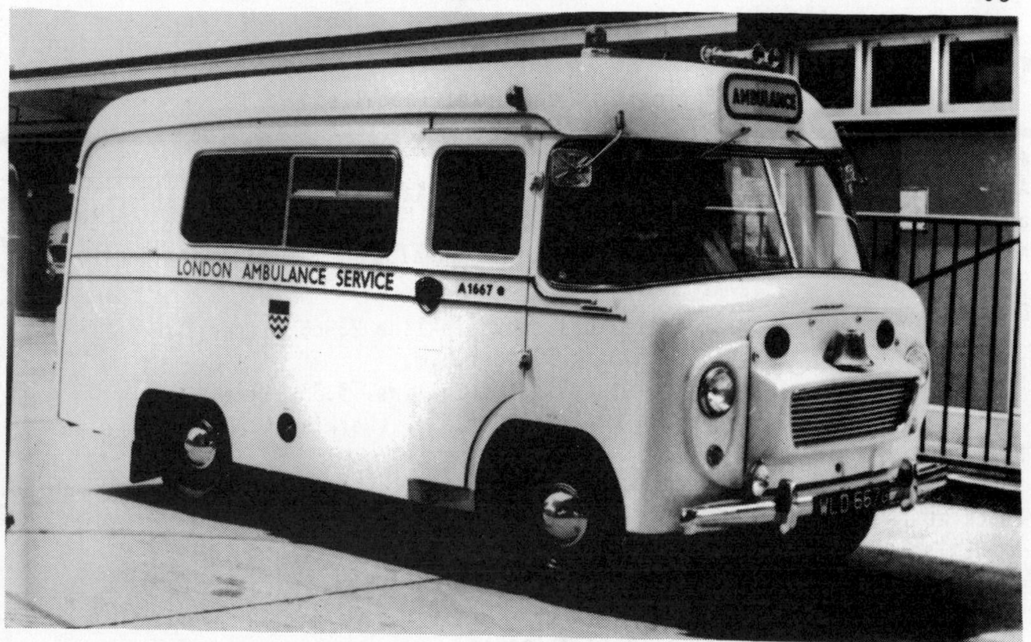

Dimensions (With Wadham Stringer body)

Overall length	4.521 m (178 inches)
Overall width	1.879 m (74 inches)
Front overhang	Not available
Rear overhang	Not available
Overall height	2.468 m (97 inches)

Weights

Chassis	Varies with equipment installed
Kerb weight	Not available

British Leyland Motor Corporation (BLMC)

Model 'FG',1970, with petrol or diesel engine. Chassis front end version, less windshield pillars and front grille. One wheelbase only.

SPECIFICATION

Engine	Petrol 4 cylinder, in-line 4.0 litre
	Diesel 4 cylinder, in-line 3.8 litre
Wheelbase	3.276 m (129 inches)
Suspension	Front & rear Semi-elliptic leaf springs
Shock absorbers	Double acting, hydraulic
Transmission	4 speed synchromesh
Tyres	7.50 x 16 10 ply

Dimensions (With Wadham Stringer body)

Overall length	5.36 m (211 inches)
Overall width	2.12 m (84 inches)
Front overhang	0.914 m (36 inches)
Rear overhang	1.143 m (45 inches)

          Overall height   2.748 m (109 inches)
Weights
          Chassis   Varies with equipment installed
          Kerb weight   3658 Kg (8066 lb)

Karrier Motors/Dennis Brothers

A combined effort between two manufacturers; Karrier, who made the chassis,
and Dennis, manufacturing the ambulance body. The chassis was based on the
Karrier/Commer 'Walk Thro' van chassis. One wheelbase. Semi-forward control.

SPECIFICATION
Engine
                            Petrol 4 cylinder, in-line 2.965 litres
                            85 b.h.p. @ 3,800 r.p.m.
                            Diesel 4 cylinder, in-line. 3.33 litre
                            63 b.h.p. @ 2,600 r.p.m. (Perkins 4.203 engine)
Wheelbase   3.124 m (123 inches)
Suspension   Front & rear Semi-elliptic leaf springs
Shock absorbers   Double acting hydraulic, telescopic f & r
Transmission   4 speed synchromesh. Manual
Tyres   7.50 x 16 8 ply.Single rear equipment
Dimensions
          Overall length   5.359 m (211 inches)
          Overall width   2.064 m (81.25 inches)
          Front overhang   Not available
          Rear overhang   Not available
          Overall height   1.778 m (70 inches)
Weights
          Chassis   2568 Kg (5656 lb) Petrol
          Kerb weight   2606 Kg (5740 lb) Diesel

Land Rover Ltd

A versatile machine capable of operating under difficult conditions and an
admirable vehicle for outlying districts, with its 4 x 4 configuration.
Chassis cab version, 4 or 6 cylinder petrol engines and a 4 cylinder diesel
engine optional equipment.

SPECIFICATION
Engine
                            Petrol 4 cylinder, in-line 2.286 litre
                            69 b.h.p. @ 4,000 r.p.m.
                            Petrol 6 cylinder, in-line 3.0 litre
                            110 b.h.p. @ 4,500 r.p.m.
                            Diesel 4 cylinder, in-line 2.286 litre
                            56.2 b.h.p. @ 4,000 r.p.m.
Wheelbase   2.77 m (109 inches)
Suspension   Front & rear Semi-elliptic leaf springs
Shock absorbers   Double acting hydraulic, telescopic, f & r
Transmission   4 speed synchromesh. Manual
Tyres   7.50 x 16 cross country tread
Dimensions (With Wadham Stringer body)
          Overall length   4.876 m (192 inches)
          Overall width   1.760 m (69 inches)

Front overhang	0.634 m (25 inches)
Rear overhang	1.45 m (57 inches)
Overall height	2.54 m (100 inches)

Weights

Chassis	Not available
Kerb weight	Not available

Another version of the Land Rover with a Wadham Stringer ambulance body is based on the chassis front end, supplied with loose cab doors and side screens, driver's and passengers' seats.

As for the Land Rover above, except –

Dimensions

Overall length	4.826 m (190 inches)
Overall width	1.760 m (69 inches)
Front overhang	0.634 m (25 inches)
Rear overhang	1.39 m (55 inches)
Overall height	2.464 m (97 inches)

<u>Range Rover</u>

4 x 4 series, 1980s, chassis front end with petrol engine, driver's and passengers' seats. The big brother to the Land Rover with a more luxurious interior. Two wheelbases offered: one standard, the second special with side loading door.

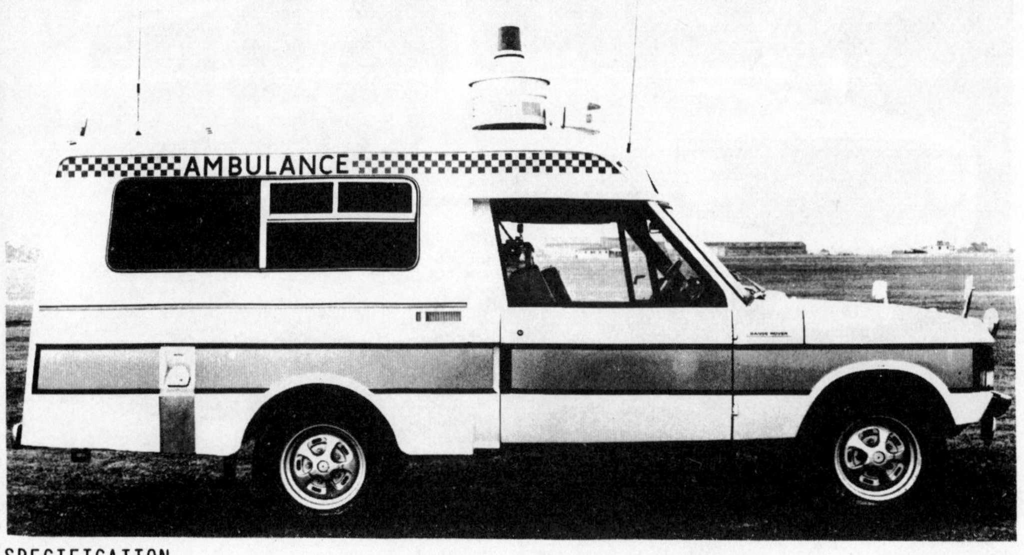

SPECIFICATION

Engine	Petrol 8 cylinder, 'V' formation. 130 b.h.p. @ 5,000 r.p.m.
Wheelbase	2.794 m (110 inches) Standard 3,429 m (135 inches) Special
Suspension	Semi-elliptic springs, front & rear
Shock absorbers	Double acting, hydraulic, telescopic f & r
Transmission	4 speed synchromesh

Tyres   205 x 16 tubed. Cross country pattern tread.
                        Single rear equipment
Dimensions (with Wadham Stringer body)
                        Standard   Special
        Overall length 5.03 m (198 inches)   5.69 m (224 inches)
        Overall width   1.803 m (71 inches)   1.803 m (71 inches)
        Front overhang 0.736 m (29 inches)   0.736 m (29 inches)
        Rear overhang   1.5 m (59 inches)   1.5 m (59 inches)
        Overall height 2.184 m (86 inches)   2.39 m (94 inches)
Weights
        Chassis   Not available
        Kerb weight   Not available

Freight/Rover (Land Rover, Ltd)

Originally Morris (Leyland) 'Sherpa'. One wheelbase. Both front and rear suspensions are single taper semi-elliptic springs giving a good ride and handling characteristics.

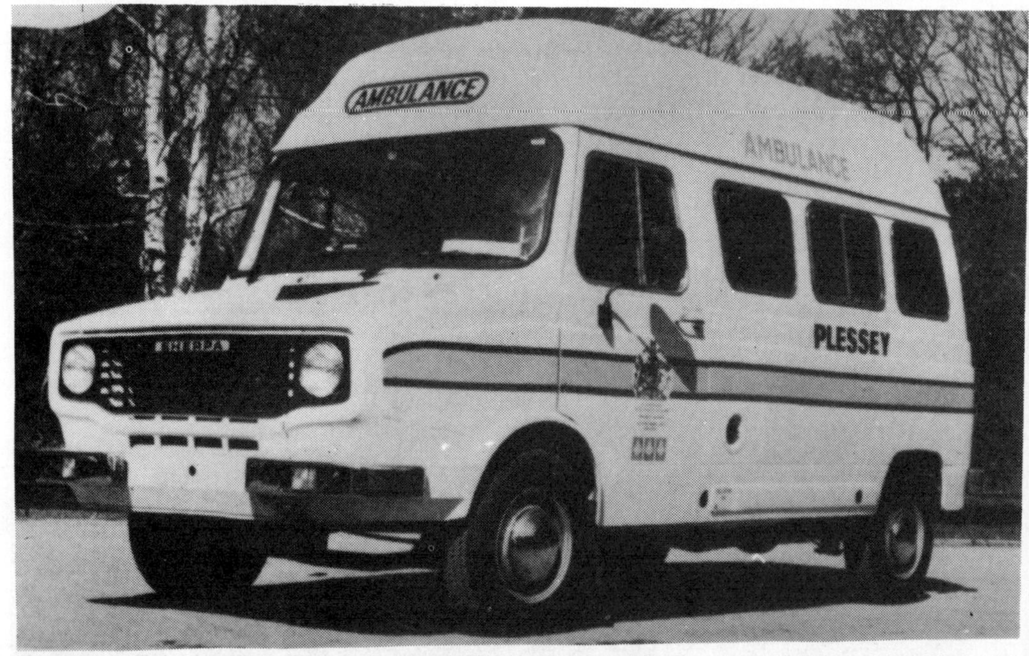

SPECIFICATION

Engine   Petrol 4 cylinder, in-line 1994 litre
                        84.5 b.h.p. @ 4,250 r.p.m.
Wheelbase   2.9 m (114 inches)
Suspension   Front & rear Single taper leaf semi-elliptic springs
Shock absorbers   Double acting hydraulic, telescopic f & r
Transmission   5 speed synchromesh. Manual
Tyres   205 x 14 6 ply rating, radial. Single rear equipment
Dimensions (With Wadham Stringer body)
        Overall length 4.95 m (194.88 inches)
        Overall width   2.02 m (79.53 inches)

Front overhang	0.9 m (35 inches)
Rear overhang	1.15 m (45.43 inches)
Overall height	Not available

Weights

Chassis	1490 Kg (3285 lb)
Kerb weight	2850 Kg (6284 lb)

Volkswagen (V.A.G. [United Kingdom] Ltd)

The Volkswagen standard van conversion by Wadham Stringer into an ambulance. One wheelbase. New 6 cylinder engine makes smoother running. Hinged cab and rear doors, single passenger seat.

SPECIFICATION

Engine	Petrol 6 cylinder, in-line 2.384 litre 90 b.h.p. @ 4,500 r.p.m.
Wheelbase	2.5 m (98.43 inches)
Suspension	Front Independent coil springs with upper & lower wishbones with a stabiliser Rear Semi-elliptic leaf springs with auxiliary rubber spring aids & Panhard rod
Shock absorbers	Double acting hydraulic, telescopic f & r
Transmission	4 speed synchromesh Manual 5 speed synchromesh Optional
Tyres	185R x 14C 8 ply rating, radial tyres.Single rear equipment

Dimensions (With Wadham Stringer body)

Overall length	4.84 m (190.55 inches)
Overall width	2.02 m (79.53 inches)
Front overhang	1.11 m (43 inches)
Rear overhang	1.23 m (48.42 inches)
Overall height	2.56 m (100.79 inches)

Weights

Chassis	2032 Kg (4480 lb)
Kerb weight	3180 Kg (7012 lb)

Talbot Motor Company Ltd.

A newcomer to the ambulance business with the conversion of their 'Express' range vans and light commercials. The ambulance conversion is on the high roof version. One wheelbase. Front wheel drive enables a low flat floor to be maintained with a low rear entrance. With independent suspension on the front of coil springs and hydraulic struts and minimum leaf semi-elliptic springs on the rear suspension with double acting hydraulic shock absorbers.

SPECIFICATION

Engine	Petrol 4 cylinder, in-line 1.971 litre 76.9 b.h.p. @ 5,000 r.p.m. (engine fitted transversely in front)
Wheelbase	3.653 m (143.8 inches)
Suspension	Front: Independent, coil springs & hydraulic struts Rear: Minimum leaf semi-elliptic springs
Shock absorbers	Double acting hydraulic, telescopic on rear only
Transmission	5 speed synchromesh. Manual

Tyres   185R x 14.Single rear equipment
Dimensions
        Overall length   4.759 m (187.4 inches)
        Overall width   1.965 m (77.4 inches)
        Front overhang   0.813 m (32 inches)
        Rear overhang   1.023 m (40.3 inches)
        Overall height   2.425 m (95½ inches)

Dodge (Karrier Motors Ltd.)

Models D953, D955 and D957 Dormobile models of the Dodge 500 range of van chassis front end versions are the base of the Social Services Welfare bus built by Dormobile, Ltd. With 2 wheelbases and 3 gross vehicle weights, both petrol and diesel engines are available.

SPECIFICATION
Engine   Diesel 4 cylinder, in-line 3.86 litre
                                79.2 b.h.p. @ 2,800 r.p.m. (Perkins U1/2)
                                Petrol 4 cylinder, in-line 2.0 litre
                                72.5 b.h.p. @ 4,300 r.p.m.
                                Diesel 6 cylinder, in-line 4.05 litres
                                93.92 b.h.p. @ 3,600 r.p.m. (Perkins Z2)
                                Petrol 6 cylinder, in-line 3.68 litres
                                88.0 b.h.p. @ 3,200 r.p.m. (Chrysler engine)
Wheelbase   3.226 m (127 inches)
                                3.658 m (144 inches)
Suspension   Front & rear Semi-elliptic leaf springs
Shock absorbers   Double acting hydraulic, telescopic f & r
Transmission   4 speed synchromesh
                                5 speed synchromesh
                                Automatic transmission (Chrysler)
Tyres   6.50R x 16 10 ply rating, for GVW of
                                4600 Kg. 8R x 17.5 tubeless optional for all GVWs
                                7.00 x 16 12 ply rating for GVW of 5600 & 6600 Kg
                                (12,348 & 14,553 lb)
Dimensions
        Overall length   4.89 m (192 in) for 3.226 m wheelbase
                                5.88 m (231 in) for 3.658 m wheelbase
        Overall width   2.046 m (80.56 inches)
        Front overhang   0.74 m (36.37 in) for 3.226 m wheelbase
        Rear overhang   1.482 m (58.35 in) for 3.658 m wheelbase
        Overall height   2.637 m (103.8 inches)
Weights   Not available (varies with model)
        GVW   4600 Kg (10,143 lb)
                                5600 Kg (12,348 lb)
                                6600 Kg (14,553 lb)

Bedford (Vauxhall Motors Ltd)

Standard Bedford 'CF' range, models 280 and 340 chassis front end and cowl versions became one of the favourites as a basic vehicle chassis for ambulance and welfare vehicle duties. One wheelbase only was offered for the Wadham Stringer Series 1X ambulance, around 1975. However, for the 1980s, Bedford introduced a series to carry 3 weight categories, models 280 and 350. Multi-role ambulance is the 3.2 metre (126 inches) wheelbase 30cwt chassis. A change to heavy duty rear springs uprates it to 35cwt. There is also a light version 25cwt chassis. An extended wheelbase of 3.7 metres (146 inches) is also available for special duties. Additional features were Quartz-halogen lights, 185 x 14 radial tyres, heavy duty alternator and twin 6 volt batteries to cope with the high electrical loads from the equipment. The General Motors automatic transmission was made available to reduce driver fatigue and give smoother running. With the full floor in the driver's compartment and the flat frame is easier for the bodybuilder to design and mount the body.

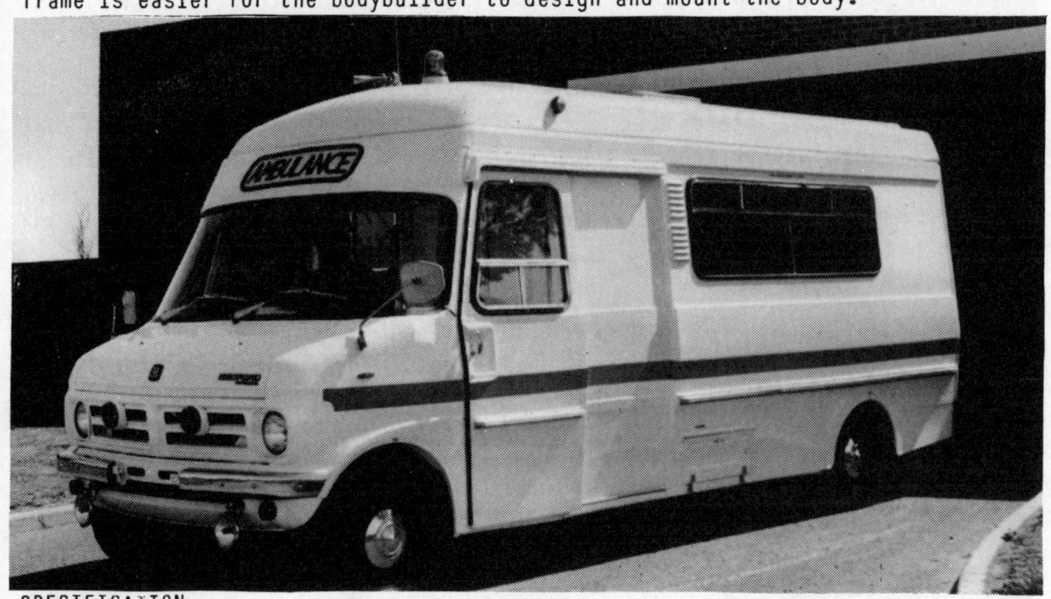

SPECIFICATION

Engine	Petrol 4 cylinder, in-line 2.3 litre
	78 b.h.p. @ 4,600 r.p.m.
Wheelbase	See above
Suspension	Front Independent coil springs
Shock absorbers	Rear Semi-elliptic leaf springs (heavy duty)
	Rear Single taper leaf semi-elliptic springs in later models
	Double acting hydraulic, telescopic f & r
Transmission	4 speed, synchromesh Manual
	Automatic transmission optional
	5 speed synchromesh Manual Optional on earlier models
Tyres	185 x 14 radial.Dual rear equipment
Dimensions	
Overall length	5.131 m (202 in) 3.22 m wheelbase
Overall width	1.981 m (78 inches)
Front overhang	0.775 m (30.5 inches)
Rear overhang	1.156 m (45.5 inches)
Overall height	2.489 m (98 inches)
	Dimensions for longer wheelbases varies with ambulance body

Weights

    Chassis
    Kerb weight   Not available
    GVW   2730 Kg (6003 lb) CF280
                         3380 Kg (7436 lb) CF340

Ford of Britain

Another popular chassis for ambulance work is the Ford Transit, models 130, 150 and 175 with Wadham Stringer ambulance body, introduced in 1970. With one wheelbase at 2.997 metres (118 inches) and using the 2.0 litre 'V' 4 petrol engine: it was replaced by the 4 cylinder in-line 2.0 litre. For the 1980s, Ford brought in a special Transit chassis front end for ambulance work, the model 160 chassis windshield version complete with a full length floor, improved suspension, fully adjustable driver's seat and provided with such items as cab doors, hinges and lock pillars and cab roof panel. This was marketed by the Special Vehicle Department of the company. Other versions of the Transit are available, such as the standard van converted by Dormobile, with a glassfibre reinforced plastic roof, increasing the interior height to 1.828 metres (72 inches).

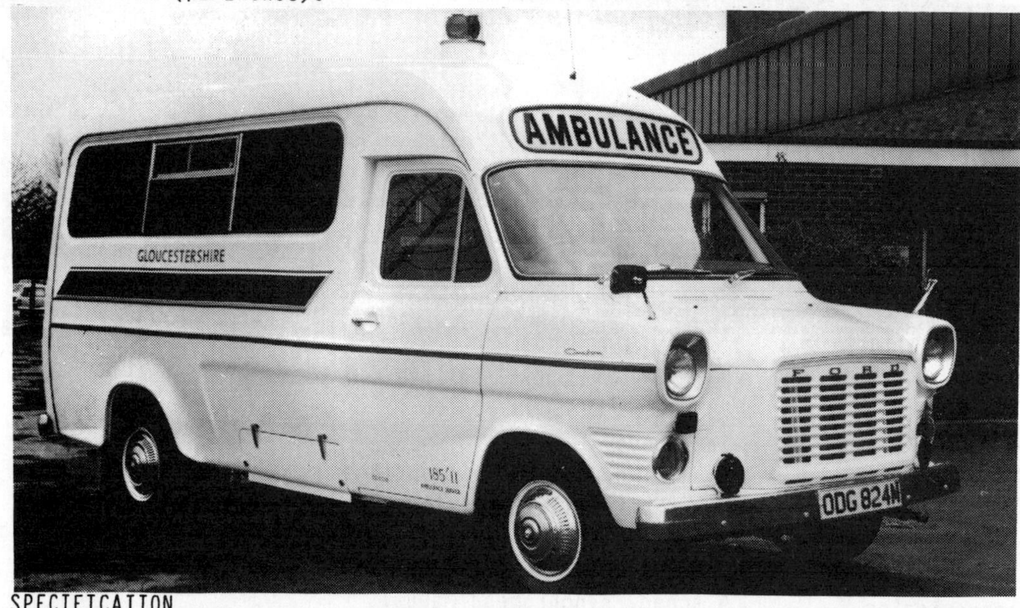

SPECIFICATION

Engine	Petrol. 4 cylinder 'V' formation 2.0 litre for older models
	Petrol 4 cylinder in-line 78 b.h.p. @ 4,500 r.p.m.
	Petrol 6 cylinder V formation 3.0 litre
	100 b.h.p. @ 4,650 r.p.m. Optional
Wheelbase	2.997 m (118 inches)
Suspension	Front & rear Minimum leaf semi-elliptic springs (1970 models)
	Single leaf tapered semi-elliptic springs (1980s)
Shock absorbers	Double acting hydraulic, telescopic f & r
Transmission	4 speed, synchromesh Manual
	Automatic transmission Optional

Tyres	185 x 14 SR.Dual rear equipment

Dimensions

Overall length	5.162 m (203 inches)
Overall width	1.981 m (78 inches)
Front overhang	0.737 m (29 inches)
Rear overhang	1.397 m (55 inches)
Overall height	2.642 m (104 inches)

Dimensions for other and later versions depend upon the design & type of ambulance or welfare vehicle body mounted.

Weights

Chassis	Not available
Kerb weight	3100 Kg (6835 lb)

<u>Transit Parcel Van</u>

The base of a conversion for a welfare ambulance. One wheelbase. A number of options are available at the customer's request. The dimensions given are those for a standard parcel body (model 160) conversion carried out by body-builders such as Wadham Stringer and Dormobile.

SPECIFICATION

Engine	Petrol 4 cylinder, in-line. 2.0 litre
	78 b.h.p. @ 4,500 r.p.m.
Wheelbase	2.997 m (118 inches)
Suspension	Front Single taper leaf semi-elliptic springs
	Rear 2 taper leaves, semi-eliptic springs
Shock absorbers	Double acting hydraulic, telescopic f & r
Transmission	4 speed synchromesh Manual
Tyres	185 x 14 radial.Dual rear equipment

Dimensions

Overall length	5.18 m (294 inches)
Overall width	2.08 m (81.8 inches)
Front overhang	0.86 m (33.8 inches)
Rear overhang	1.32 m (52 inches)
Overall height	2.64 m (104 inches)

Weights

Chassis	1648 Kg (3633 lb)
Kerb weight	3265 Kg (7200 lb)

<u>'A' Series</u>

The 2 standard models, A0609 and A0610 at 3.96 metres (156 inches) wheelbase, are good basic chassis windshield versions for welfare buses, specially adapted for the carriage of invalid wheelchair patients. Such additional equipment as heavy duty batteries and alternator to cope with the increased electrical lead from the equipment. There is available a high centre of gravity package to improve stability. Two versions are available, one with hinged door for the driver and a jacknife type for the front entrance on the nearside, the other with sliding doors on both sides.

SPECIFICATION

Engine	Diesel 6 cylinder, in-line. 3.5 litre
	89 b.h.p. @ 3,600 r.p.m. [A0609]
	Petrol 6 cylinder, 'V' formation 3.0 litre
	100 b.h.p. @ 4,500 r.p.m. [A0610]
Wheelbase	3.96 m (156 inches)
Suspension	Semi-elliptic leaf springs
Shock absorbers	Front, 6 leaves; Rear 3 leaves
Transmission	Double acting, hydraulic, Telescopic f & r
	4 speed synchromesh. Manual
Tyres	7.00 x 16 12 ply rating. Dual rear equipment
	7.50 x 16 12 ply rating Optional
	Radial tyres also available as optional
Dimensions	(with body by Dormobile)
Overall length	7.226 m (284 inches) max.
Overall width	2.2 m (86 inches) approx.
Front overhang	0.89 m (35 inches)
Rear overhang	2.376 m (93 inches) max.
Overall height	Not available
Weights	
Chassis	Not available
Kerb weight	6300 Kg (13891 lb) Diesel
	6100 Kg (13450 lb) Petrol

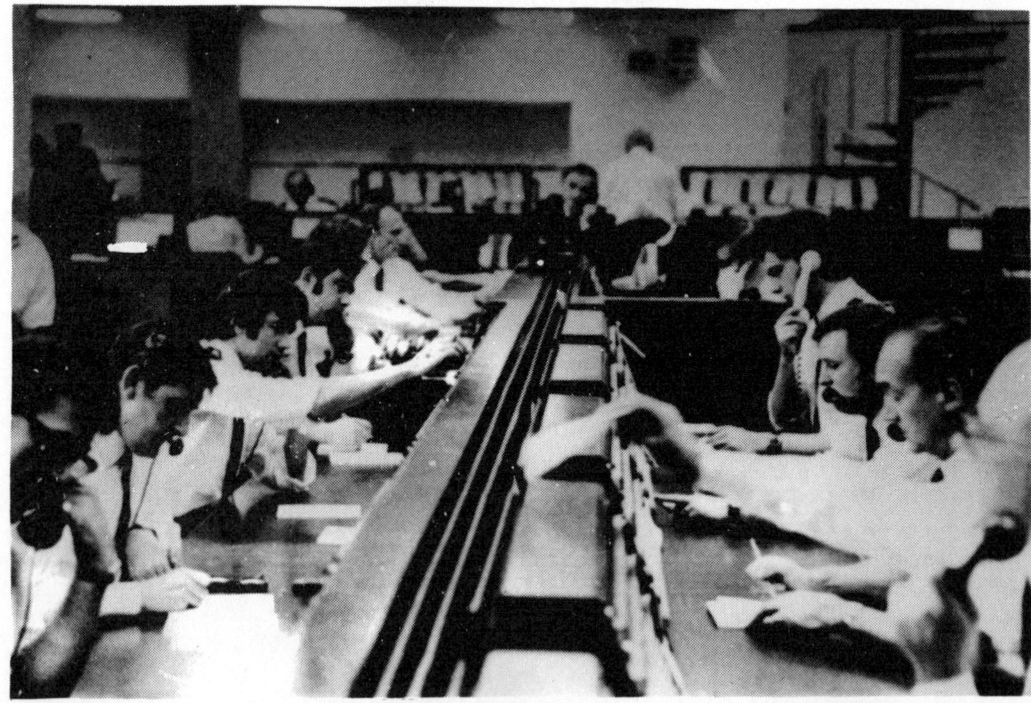

London Ambulance Service Headquarters Control

(by permission of London Ambulance Service)

Operational Control

The aim of a control must always be to keep a fleet of ambulances as effectively operational as possible. This can be done only with quick and reliable methods of communication between the Control and the Ambulance: to achieve this each ambulance is equipped with mobile radio transceivers.

One of the most important systems in dealing with emergencies is this radio control, enabling flexibility of the ambulances, moving them to areas where heavy pressure of incidents occur and in helping to transfer patients without undue delay.

The London Ambulance Service Control is a typical example of a first class operational system -

In the Greater London area 15 ambulance controls were operational in 1965. In 1972 this number was reduced to 6 when the new Central Ambulance Control opened. These 6 were - Central Ambulance Control, the Inner Zone Control, (both these located at the London Headquarters in Waterloo Road) and four Local Divisional Controls.

The Central Ambulance Control covers all emergency calls and non-urgent patients who are stretcher cases, while the Inner Zone Control is responsible for organising transport of outpatients to and from a number of major hospitals in Inner London drawing patients from the whole of London. It also deals with routine transport for outpatients living in the five Inner Boroughs.

The 4 Local Controls deal with routine transport for sitting cases as outpatients.

Each is situated in one of the divisions where the service is separated for the purposes of ambulance and station management. The Control is kept in touch with the ambulance and can, with a 'selecting calling' system call any specific ambulance automatically. This is achieved by punching the ambulance's individual callsign on to digital buttons arranged on the Control's radio panel. This makes a light in the selected vehicle flash continually until one of the crew radios back to Control. Similarly, the ambulance crew can radio Control by simply depressing the transmitting button when the ambulance callsign is displayed on the Control radio panel.

A new contact aid called the 'Automatic Vehicle Updating' is being brought into use. With the new system a radio, complete with a panel of knobs, is fitted in the ambulance. By pushing the appropriate knob the driver is automatically able to transmit to the Control the identity of his vehicle and the current state of availability - that is, whether it has arrived and still at the scene of an accident; if the ambulance is going to the hospital; or, operation completed, is returning to Control.

This information is shown on an ambulance availability map at the Control Room. The advantage is that the ambulance crew or driver is no longer required to keep in constant touch by speech to Control as to the vehicle's whereabouts.

There are 3 sections in a divisional control - future bookings, planning and movement. Requests for ambulances, stretcher or sitting cases, are received in many ways; by means of a letter from a doctor or other authorised person specifying the dates when travelling assistance is needed, by telephone and by telex (generally for urgent cases) and by hand for urgent cases, specific dates or immediate attention.

At the Control the planning section prepares requests for transport for the day, and future dates, all based on the information collected by the future booking team, who feed all relevant information into the computer. Routes are prepared to make the most economical use of the ambulances available and these also take into account the variety of the patients' disabilities, their home addresses, times of appointment and hospitals to be visited. These are prepared and fed into the computer which spells out how patients can be dealt with - some together in one journey, some where two or three journeys are necessary - and shows up the daily programme, as well as co-ordinating programmes for the following days.

The National Health Service Act of 1977 directed the Secretary of State to provide ambulance services to meet all reasonable requirements considered necessary. This Service was passed to the Area Health Authorities, except in metropolitan counties, where the Service became the responsibilty of the Regional Health Authorities.

The ambulance service has to provide suitable transport, normally to the nearest hospital, but can go to any other hospital for special treatment or because of the availability of beds for more urgent cases, if the patient is medically unfit to travel by any other method, that is public transport, private transport (either their own, relations' or friends' or voluntary services) and also being able to walk.

The responsibility for requesting an ambulance and its destination is that of the doctor, midwife or dentist, but in emergency any person can ask for an ambulance through the 999 call, which covers accidents anywhere or sudden illness in public places. Place, time, and possibly medical details to assist the ambulance control should be given. Under these circumstances an ambulance must be available immediately, even if it means contacting other Controls outside the area.

Not all ambulance availability is limited to the N.H.S; it is possible to call on an ambulance to carry patients to and from private nursing homes and hospitals on the same terms and conditions as for the N.H.S. patients, providing the length of the journey involved is no longer than travelling to the nearest general hospital. A private patient can be taken to a private hospital further away, providing that it is not detrimental to any N.H.S. patient; however, the actual cost of the extra mileage involved may have to be paid. But if it is against the benefit of other patients to use N.H.S. ambulances for this purpose, the private patient must make other arrangements.

National Health Service ambulances and crews may be provided to supplement the voluntary ambulance services at sporting or other public events, where accidents or emergencies may warrant such assistance. In this case, written undertakings are made in advance. Payment is a matter for the discretion of the Authorities, depending upon circumstances.

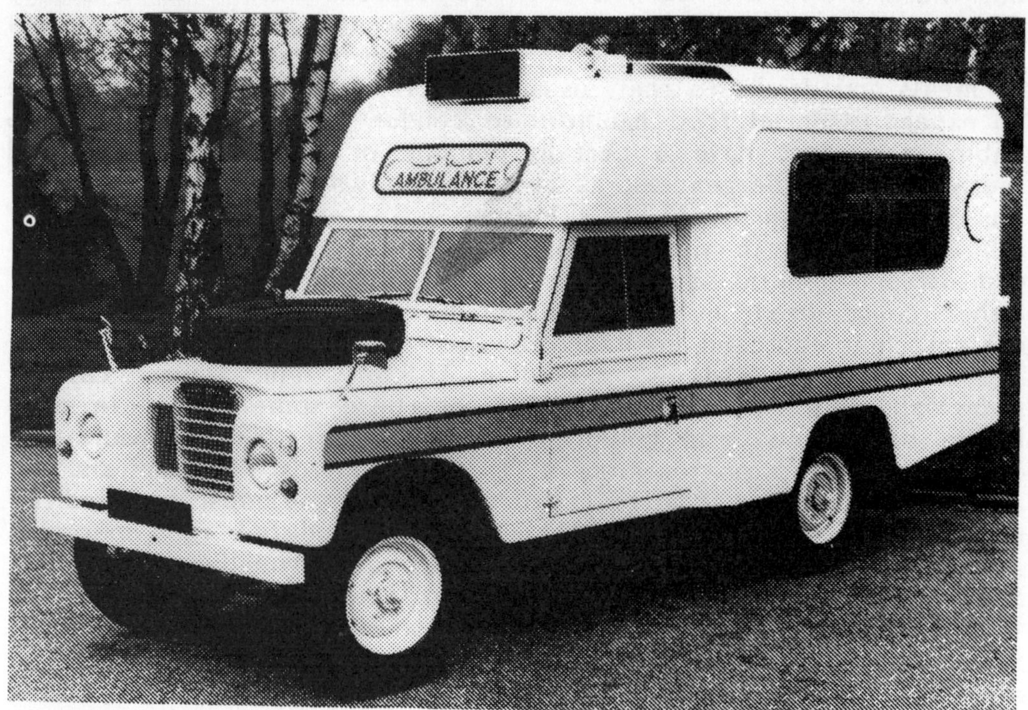

Land Rover ambulance with Wadham Stringer body , 1980s

Air Ambulances

Commercial airlines cannot carry invalid passengers on normal scheduled flights to the detriment of its services to the normal travelling public. For instance, an airline will not accept cases where behaviour or appearance is disturbing or could be offensive to other passengers. The public have their rights to be protected from such situations, particularly when the patient is offensive in any way.

Sometimes there is a general assumption that the aircraft cabin crew can give nursing facilities and aids, including toileting, but these crews are carried for two reasons only – as a safety measure to open and close aircraft doors and evacuate the passenger cabins in an emergency and to provide a service in the form of meals and drinks to their passengers. It is therefore unreasonable to expect essential food handlers to conduct nursing activities. The cabin crew does have a certain amount of training in first aid measures and emergencies, as there can always be times when a passenger is taken ill during a journey.

Therefore, in view of the average air passenger expecting comfort and general service, it is essential that special aircraft be either constructed as or converted to air ambulances with the correct equipment and medical crew.

The world airlines, excluding U.S.S.R. and China, carried some 650 million passengers in 1979: of these some 10% were sick, infirm or disabled and could be travelling for early consultation opinion, diagnosis or treatment at medical centres and hospitals.

The first use of aircraft for ambulance use must be credited to the French around 1920, when they considered the operation seriously for the evacuation of the sick and wounded from their Middle East possessions. The aircraft used was a modified Breguet 14T, a civilian plane version of the standard French Army Air Service operational reconnaissance and day bomber single engined aircraft.

Accommodation was in the fuselage between the engine and the cockpit and stretchers were placed one above the other. The after part of the sides of the cabin could be quickly removed to accept the stretchers, the upper stretcher being inserted first and swung into position by wires passing over pulleys, while the lower one was placed underneath on the floor of the aircraft. Full complement was two stretchers and one sitting case. Electrically heated warming bags were provided for the stretchers, as was a supply of oxygen, first aid equipment, bed pans and urine bottle. The average speed was around 85 m.p.h.

An older type of air ambulance, superseded by the 14T, was a modified Breguet 14A2, the pilot of which was in front, with the two strechers placed behind in the fuselage. It had comparitive exposure and very limited space in the absence of a purpose-built cabin. The only other type in existence at that time were two seaplanes modified for ambulance use at French naval stations.

This air service proved successful when, in 1922, 1,200 wounded were evacuated from Morocco and the Levant during activities in those areas.

However, from the experience gained by the French medical authorities, Great Britain took up the idea and it is believed that the Royal Air Force used the first air ambulance in British overseas territories and, later, in GreatBritain. The first British air ambulance, built in 1920 for the R.A.F., was based on a Vickers Vernon twin engined aircraft: to load the stretchers a hatch door in the front nose of the plane was opened and they were passed through this down a tunnel which opened up into the interior of the fuselage. Collapsible stretcher racks in two tiers along one side of the fuselage, took 4 stretchers with separate regulated oxygen supply for each. Wash basin, electric kettle, heated body warmers, cupboards for medical supplies and drugs, and a screened-off water closet in the rear of the aircraft were included. Light and ventilation was also given. After a few modifications and adjustments, the plane was dismantled and sent to Aboukir, Egypt, in 1922 to be re-assembled there; unfortunately, this first air ambulance crashed and was completely beyond repair. Two similar ambulances were built, but with some modifications - the oxgyen apparatus was simplified; the wash basin was removed; 2 lower stretchers were taken out; 10 folding deck chairs were introduced, 6 under the upper stretchers and 4 on the opposite side of the fuselage, these proving very comfortable for patients who would have been semi-stretcher cases; there were other modifications on windows, including ventilation.

Again, these aircraft were dispatched to Aboukir, re-assembled and put into service. One crashed on its way to Baghdad in the latter part of 1922, but it was repairable. The other flew many successful missions. In 1924 more air ambulances were being re-assembled at Aboukir, all of the same type.

In 1923 a new single-engined aircraft, the Avro Andover air ambulance, was built, 3 being commissioned in Great Britain by

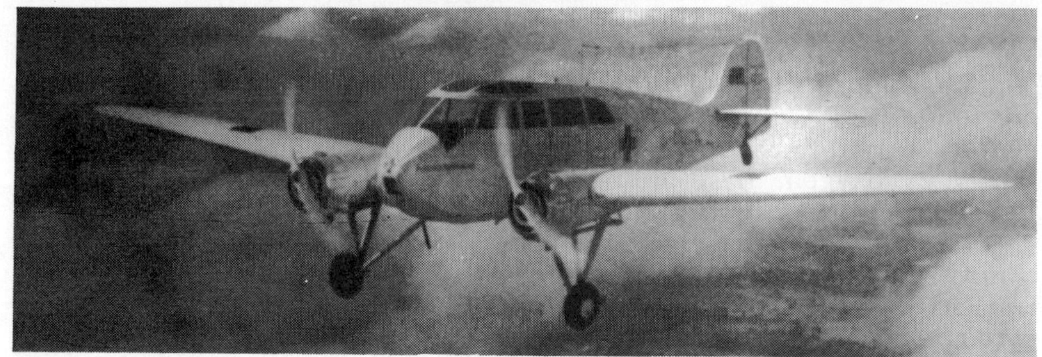

A British Red Cross Society air ambulance, 1930s

1925. It had space for 2 stretchers and 2 sitting cases, or 4 sitting cases. Stretchers were loaded through the side door in the fuselage. The seats were in canvas and of the folding type similar to the Vickers Vernon. It was an improvement in several ways - it had greater headroom, approximately 6 feet; ventilation by exhaust fan in the rear of the fuselage, a regulated supply of hot air being taken in from outside of the exhaust pipe; it had a petrol capacity of 7 hours flight with full load.

This machine was particularly suitable, as its accommodation was sufficient for the demand, if run regularly, to cope with an average number of casualties. It was also useful for emergency work and routine evacuation of the sick and injured from outlying places, on which work it had been tried in England, although it was not practical for any large scale evacuation.

The Vernon Victoria was better for the carriage of large numbers of casualties. Similar to the Vickers Vernon, it was used as a troop carrier for 24 passengers. With 2 stretcher racks and folding deck chairs to carry 12 sitting cases, the Vernon Victoria could take 14 casualties and, additionally, have 2 stretchers on extra floor space when necessary. It was an admirable air ambulance for mass evacuation and had the advantage of being a standard type available in numbers if needed for medical work.

Another type of air ambulance used by the Royal Navy - more like a single special stretcher carrier - was associated with the Neill Robertson stretcher, used by the Navy for transhipping invalid patients. The stretcher consisted of a piece of green canvas, with strengthening bamboo battens on the outside. Webbing straps with buckles were attached to the canvas to totally strap the patient on to the stretcher. Rope slings were put on to the battens to lower the stretcher from ships, these straps being retained as a ready means of securing the stretcher to the aircraft fuselage. In addition, a head pillow was strapped to the interior surface of the stretcher. A one-piece cover of green canvas, lined with blanketing (similar to a monk's habit - cloak and cowl) and provided with press-studs to take a second lining if needed. With the patient well strapped up, placed on the stretcher, this cover completely encased both, the lined flap extending from the back was folded over and secured to protect the patient's feet. Finally a face mask was provided for the patient - and it appeared that he would really need it! The whole apparatus was put on the top of the fuselage of either a 2 seater De Haviland 9A or a Bristol fighter. Attachment to the aircraft was by each of 6 grommet loops on the stretcher supplied with a 1 inch wide leather strap: the upper 4 were 14 inches long and the lower 2 36 inches long. A canvas strap, 4 inches wide, encircled the fuselage, connected to the foot ring on the stretcher by a 36 inch long strap to stop lateral movement of the apparatus during flight. Each strap was clearly marked as to its function in the attachment.

Specifications of the Original Air Ambulances
These were the aircraft used by the Royal Air Force for ambulance work during the 1920s, including the French Breguet 14T aerial ambulance -

Vickers-Vernon 1st type

Engines	Twin engines. 450 h.p. Napier Lion
Maximum speed	$119\frac{1}{2}$ m.p.h.
Touring speed	90 m.p.h.
Landing speed	50 m.p.h.
Fuel capacity	4 hours
Dimensions of cabin-	
Length	5.18 m (204 inches)
Height	1.83 m (72 inches)
Width	1.12 m (44 inches)
Communications	Radio: air & ground
Accommodation	4 stretchers
Crew	2 pilots, 1 wireless operator, 1 orderly, 1 fitter

Special features   Oxygen to all stretchers; Electrically lit; electric body warmers & kettle; wash-basin & W.C.; ventilation by electric fan in forward bulk-head & ventilators in rear; Triplex glass windows; stretcher cases loaded through nose of machine.

Vickers Vernon 2nd type

Specification similar to 1st type except for -

Accommodation   2 stretcher and up to 10 sitting cases, depending on distance to be travelled and size of crew.

Special features   10 special folding chairs, also used by the non-pilot crew; ventilation from the slip stream of the propeller through hinged forward windows; window gauze throughout.

Vernon Victoria

Specification similar to Vickers Vernon, except for

Fuel capacity   9 hours

Accommodation   2 stretcher and between 10 and 12 sitting cases, depending on distance to be travelled and size of crew.

Special features   6 double folding chairs looking sideways. Transparent wind-proof windows. Stretcher cases loaded through nose of machine.

Avro Andover

Engine	Single 650 h.p. Rolls Condor, with auxiliary starting motor
Maximum speed	106 m.p.h.
Touring speed	85 m.p.h.
Landing speed	50 m.p.h.
Dimensions of cabin –	
Length	5.48 metres (216 inches)
Height	1.83 m (72 inches)
Width	1.42 m (56 inches)
Communications	Radio
Fuel capacity	7 hours
Accommodation	2 stretchers, up to 4 sitting cases
Crew	Pilot, Wireless operator, Orderly
Special features	The 2 stretcher racks, when in use, take the place of the 2 rear folding chairs; Triplex glass windows; ample locker space for kits, etc.; heating from outside of exhaust pipe; electric kettle; W.C.

Breguet 14T

Engine	Single 300 h.p. Renault
Maximum speed	199 m.p.h.
Touring & landing speeds	Not available
Fuel capacity	$4\frac{1}{2}$ hours
Dimensions of cabin	–
Length	2.08 m (82 inches)
Height	1.44 m (57 inches)
Width	1.04 m (40 inches)
Communications	None
Accommodation	2 stretchers, 1 sitting case
Crew	1 pilot
Special features	Oxygen supplied to both stretcher cases; electrically heated blankets; ventilation under complete control

The Royal Air Force studied the situation and as a result, it was decided that the various aircraft could play a part in future conflicts –

For single casualties: perhaps the Neill Robertson modified stretcher apparatus could by considered invaluable.

Single engined air ambulances capable of taking one stretcher case and 2 sitting cases could be developed and be a part of every 2/3 seater squadron.

The Avro Andover type was ideal for routine evacuation of invalids. The new Vernon troop carrier aircraft, modified to air ambulance as and when required, was necessary for the evacuation of casualties on a large scale.

During this time no organised service, as such, was operating in the British Isles. Again, the military (all services) were the first priority, as that originally given to the motor ambulance.

Probably the first organised civilian service was the Scottish Air Ambulance Service, providing a link between the outlying parts of the country with the hospitals. Today this service covers a network of 45 islands and Highlands airstrips to and from the mainland airports.

It started in 1933 when Dr Stewart in the Scottish island of Islay, attending a patient, a 33-year-old fisherman, John McDermid, found that he was suffering from perforations of the stomach, meaning that peritonitis was a real threat and that it was essential to get him to hospital for surgery. The crossing to the mainland by boat would take 10 hours and then there would be the road journey to the hospital, but time was not on McDermid's side. The alternative was to find an aircraft to fly the patient across to the mainland. Dr Stewart telegraphed the St Andrew's Ambulance Association for help in finding an aircraft to take his patient to the Western Infirmary at Glasgow for urgent surgery. The Association contacted the Scottish Flying Club at Renfrew Airport, near Glasgow. Midland & Scottish Air Ferries, stationed there, had recently taken delivery of two aircraft fitted out as flying ambulances - twin engined De Haviland 84 Dragon Moths. Half an hour after the Association had received the telegram, a pilot took off for Islay. 45 minutes later he landed on the sands at Lochindaal and received the patient, together with a nurse, and flew back to Renfrew, where a motor ambulance was waiting to rush John McDermid off to Glasgow. The total time from despatch of the telegram to admission to hospital was $4\frac{1}{4}$ hours.

The first air ambulance flight from the Isle of Skye took place two months after John McDermid's ordeal. This was another dramatic incident. Dr Fothergill was taken ill whilst on holiday at Uig. An aircraft from Midland & Scottish Air Ferries went into operation once more, landed at Kilmuir, 5 miles south of the town. The patient, with his wife and doctor, were taken aboard and flown to the Royal Infirmary at Edinburgh. The journey was a very eventful one, amidst thunder, lightning and torrential rain; the aircraft was almost forced down, but managed to continue flying low to the airfield. Dr Fothergill was safely admitted to the infirmary.

The newspapers got to work spreading these stories throughout Scotland. Within a short time the ambulance service had been extended to Kintyre, islands in the Hebrides and to the Northern Islands. Midland & Scottish Air Ferries continued to operate the service, also using a Fox Moth aircraft and, from 1935 onwards, a Spartan Cruiser.

It was such flights through the years that built up the Scottish Air Ambulance Service and, by 1945, something like 100 patients and 20,000 miles a year were being achieved.

British European Airways took over the air ambulance operation in 1947. The De Haviland Rapide was used for the service,

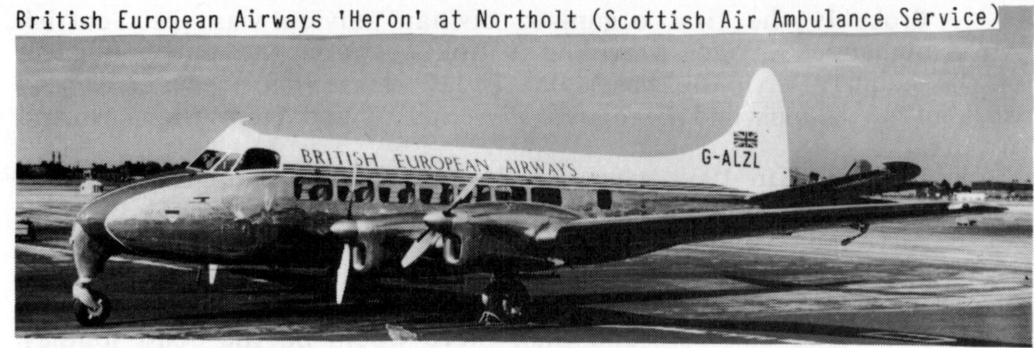

British European Airways 'Heron' at Northolt (Scottish Air Ambulance Service)

with occasional assistance from a DC 3 aircraft until 1955. Later a change was made and four engined D.H. Herons replaced the Rapide.

The two De Haviland Herons 1B aircraft at the time being used on certain internal routes in Scotland were easily converted into air ambulances. It involved removing the seats and fitting a specially designed stretcher unit with all necessary equipment and oxygen supply sets. The nursing equipment was stored in the lockers beneath the stretcher rack. The DC 3 still stood by for ambulance duties in case the Herons were not immediately available because of maintenance or repair.

A great change came in 1948 on the formation of the National Health Service. Loganair, Ltd., a small but successful commercial air service in Scotland, came to share the operation with S.A.A.S. and B.E.A. from 1965 to 1973, after which it took over the entire operation.

For a long time De Haviland had provided all the aircraft for the air ambulance business. However, as the service grew and spread its wings further afield during the 60s, these D H Heron aircraft had difficulty in landing on some of the island airstrips, which were too short for the planes' landing procedure. The Secretary of State for Scotland in the early 70s investigated the problem and declared that the Heron was unsuitable for general ambulance service and so recommended to the N.H.S. that other makes or types of aircraft should be researched and bought. Consequently, Loganair introduced another aircraft, the Britten Norman Islander, a well-established and reliable machine designed and developed for service to the Scottish islands.

For many years now the national organisations have worked together on the Scottish Air Ambulance Service – the Scottish Home & Health Department (the Scottish branch of the N.H.S.) is responsible for the funds for the service, while the fee for the airline operating the service is negotiable on an annual basis.

For the past 11 years Loganair, providing specially trained men and aircraft for the S.A.A.S. has proved a very successful and effective operation.

In the early days the nurses had been supplied by Paisley Nursing Association, the payment being one guinea (£1.05): the nurse who accompanied John McDermid on that first flight in 1933 just happened to be on holiday in Islay at the time. From 1942 onwards the Southern General Hospital in Glasgow took over the responsibility of providing nurses: 8 volunteers, all over 24 years old, complete with packed bag, formed the S.A.A.S. squad. In the 1960s the hospital provided a roster of 75 trained nurses, on call day and night for air ambulance duties. These nurses were trained in aviation medical attention and care and given a thorough briefing at Loganair base on safety equipment and procedures. As a travelling nurse, she will be briefed in advance on the details of the patient she is to accompany to the hospital and will also be selected for a particular medical problem in which she may have had experience and she is likely to be looking after the patient during the hospital treatment.

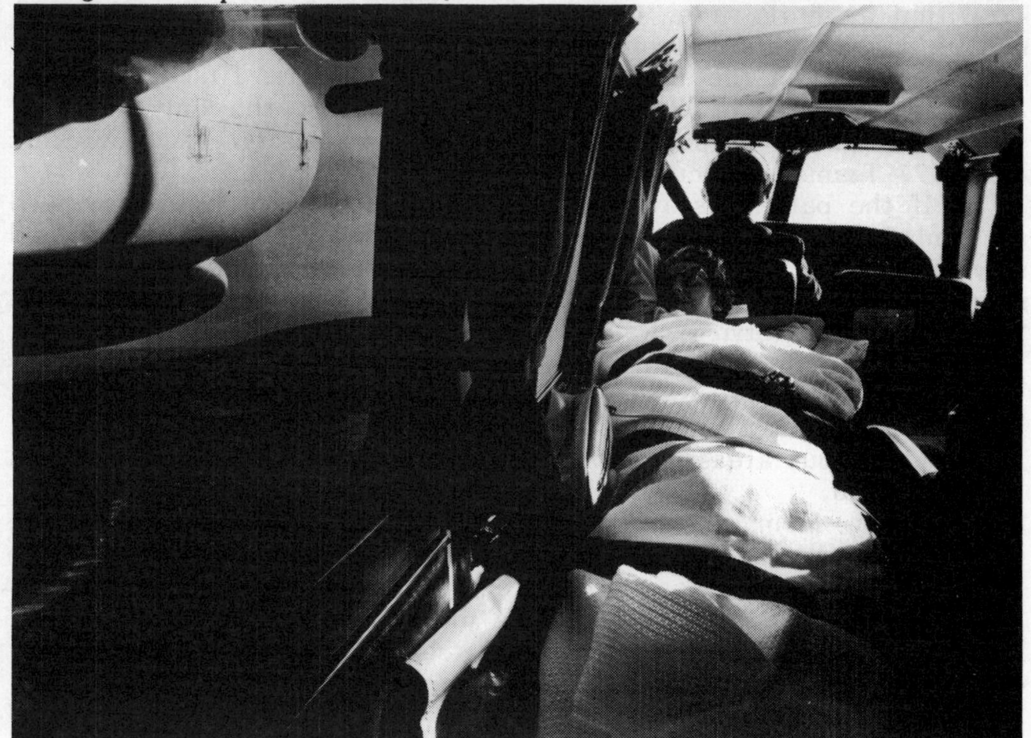

Interior of Loganair Air Ambulance

In addition these nurses have to carry out emergency survival drills on a yearly basis.

The following is the code of practice used for getting the services of the S.A.A.S. –

1. The doctor who wants the air ambulance service for speed in getting a patient to hospital for treatment takes the following action.

2. He telephones or telegraphs the mainland hospital and fixes a bed for the patient: the same procedure as a mainland doctor.
3. He calls the Operations Officer at Glasgow, Lerwick or Kirkwall and makes the air ambulance booking.
4. Loganair take down all details, referring to any infection, special treatment necessary, drugs required and administered during the flight.
5. Loganair then sets in motion the system to get the aircraft refuelled, loaded and ready for flight. The nurse(s) are alerted and a taxi arranged to pick her, or them, up to transport them to the airport. The hospital is told of the return flight time to have an ambulance ready at the airfield to get the patient, the nurse, and maybe the doctor, to the hospital.
6. Within a short time of the call being received from the doctor, Loganair can have an air ambulance with pilot and nurse or nurses on the tarmac ready to leave.
7. Within a short time, depending upon the distance, the patient can be admitted into hospital.

Apart from the usual stretcher racks, seats, first aid equipment and stowage of drugs and medical items, the only item of special equipment purpose built for use in an aircraft is a Vickers Model 77 Transport Incubator.

If the patient is at a place unsuitable for the normal winged air ambulance to operate, he or she is picked up by an armed services helicopter, usually an S55, and taken to the nearest landing strip to be transferred to the waiting air ambulance. The Scottish Air Ambulance Service, in association with Royal Navy and Royal Air Force helicopters, provides a very efficient and widespread network to cover all the widely scattered rural and island districts with a population of some 60,000 people. Some distances, over sea and mountainous areas, can be as much as 180 to 200 miles from a large hospital.

Apart from carrying urgent cases to hospitals, there are occasions when the air ambulance flies out specialists to remote areas where their services are urgently needed, with the possibility of taking any patient found wanting urgent attention to the nearest hospital. Many patients return home by the service, saving long overland and/or sea journeys.

When the record of the Scottish Air Ambulance Service and of Logan is considered, operating through all kinds of weather day and night, in and out of remote areas, saving hundreds of lives, travelling thousands of miles during this last 50 years, with only one fatal accident, it is nothing less than fantastic.

In the mid-30s it was possible to charter an aircraft fitted out as an ambulance to take patients to hospitals at various destinations. These were to be chartered from Imperial Airways at Croydon Airport. This was when more and more doctors were

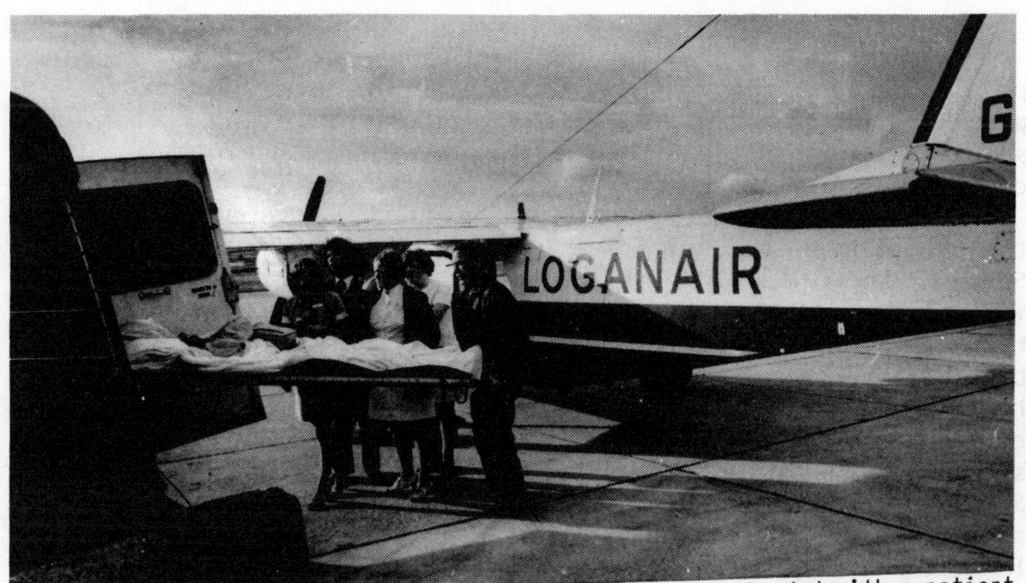

Air Ambulance being loaded with a patient

recommending the use of aircraft for ambulance work, where patients in critical conditions had to be taken to hospitals in the shortest possible time. In such cases, doctors could hire from Imperial Airways an air ambulance equipped for smooth and swift carriage of patients: within these aircraft there was ample room for a doctor and a nurse to accompany the patient if needed.

One particular incident was in October, 1934, when a doctor was faced with the problem of getting a young patient from London to Zurich, Switzerland, for treatment. The child was in a weak condition having had one thigh amputated for extensive osteo-myelitis and it was decided that the only way the journey could be made was by air. Imperial Airways were approached and arrangements were made to reserve and convert the forward cabin of one of their latest types of four engined aircraft. This cabin usually held 10 passengers, so the backs of 4 seats were removed and a wooden bed, 6 feet by 3 feet, was erected, complete with Dunlopillo mattress; also in the cabin were the doctor, a male nurse and the patient's mother. The patient was taken from a nursing home in West London at 7 a.m. to Croydon Airport and lifted directly from the motor ambulance bed to that in the aircraft. The journey started at 8.05, reaching Zurich at 2.15 p.m. (half an hour stop at Paris and a quarter of an hour at Basle). At Zurich an ambulance was waiting to take the patient to the hospital where he was admitted at precisely 3.15 and laid as comfortably as possible in bed.

At that time Imperial Airways also had smaller special charter aircraft, with three engines, containing a full length bed and accommodation for two other people, which could be hired at

1s.6d (7½p.) a mile.

In the late 50s it was proposed that helicopters could help or perhaps replace the existing fixed wing aircraft, but, except for possible link-ups to islands possessing airstrips, it was not considered feasible due to the adverse weather conditions often encountered in remote areas.

One service that started in March, 1979, is associated with the oil fields in the North Sea: it is the Bristow Search and Rescue Service. Their Bell 212 Model helicopters, twin bladed rotor, are well-tried machines and ideal for sea-air rescue (S.A.R.) Six of these helicopters, with equipment - stretchers, morphine, sleeping bags, winches and hoists - can be housed on the 'Treasure Finder' hanger rig in the Brent Field in the North Sea. Various units of equipment have been developed by Bristow in conjunction with specialist manufacturers: one such is the Forward Looking Infra-Red Scanner (F.L.I.R.), designed to enable a helicopter crew locate a survivor in the sea without actually having to 'see' him. The F L I R detects temperature from the survivor's body in the form of infra-red transmissions which are then displayed on a T.V. monitor in the helicopter. At 2,000 feet the scanner can detect a temperature difference as slight as 0.2 of a degree centigrade and would produce an image on the screen, where the survivor's head would show up clearly against the colder water. With an auto-hover system combined with the F L I R, the rescue helicopter crew can locate a survivor and then with their computer work out a flight pattern to bring the helicopter over the survivor. The medic is then lowered to the sea to rescue the casualty. Bristow also offer assistance when requested with their Hawker-Siddeley HS 125 700 aircraft fitted with a stretcher and medical equipment.

Another system introduced by this company for night sea searches is 'Night Sun' - a giant helicopter-mounted 65 million candlepower arclight unique in the helicopter world. Its 300 foot focussable beam, operated by joystick by the co-pilot, is designed to overcome the problems of poor visability. A second machine flies in tandem with the helicopter carrying the arclight to help in the search and rescue.

The St John's Ambulance Association formed an Air Wing in 1972. Initially to speed limited-life organs, such as kidneys and livers, from one hospital to another for transplant operations by using lightweight aircraft, the Wing also delivers urgently needed medical supplies. All personnel are volunteers, as are the other divisions of the St John. Currently the Air Wing has 175 pilots and 105 aircraft ready for any emergency and on call 24 hours a day. At the Air Wing centres the traffic is directed by 13 controllers, volunteers, who aim to have any aircraft airborne within one hour of any emergency call being received. To call the service requests go from individuals to the Department of Health Transport Service, Bristol; these are then routed to Flight Control Centre at St

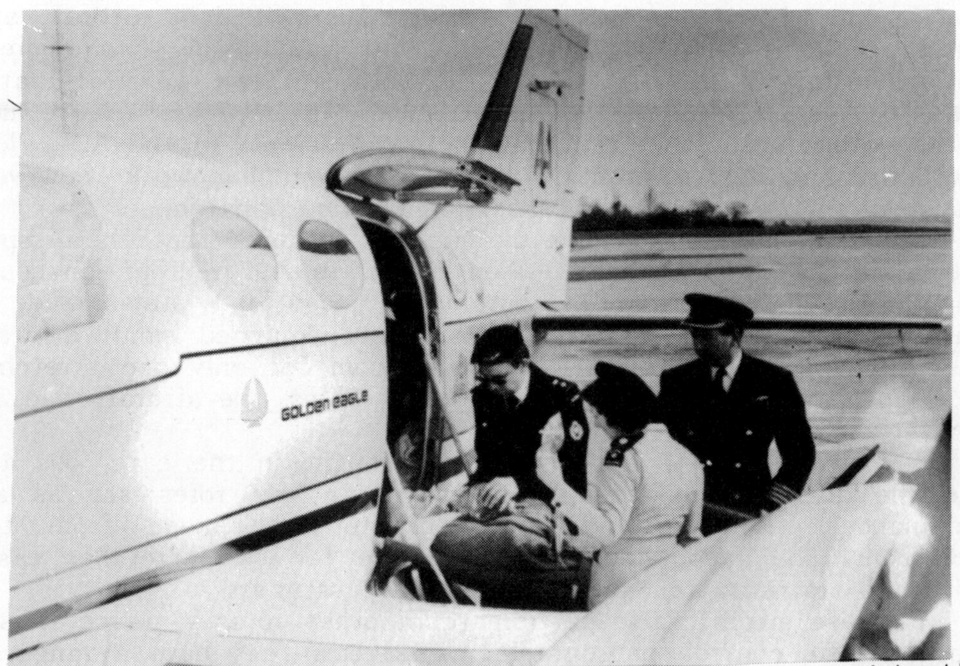

St John Ambulance air attendants transfer a patient from an Automobile
Association ambulance plane after a repatriation flight from overseas
(by permission of St John Ambulance Association)

Margaret's Hospital, Epping, Essex. As soon as an organ becomes available and is matched to a waiting patient, the organ is on its way to the nearest airfield and, whilst this journey is being made, the final destination and flight arrengements are given to Flight Control.

There are similar organ matching centres in France, Netherlands, Belgium, Germany and Scandinavia, which are linked to the computer in Great Britain.

The St John Ambulance Air Wing has made 406 journeys covering 250,000 miles. Co-operation has been given by the Royal Air Force, the Royal Navy and Civil Aviation Authorities in providing assistance to better the operation. In addition to the Air Wing, a branch known as Aeromedical Services, which is the air ambulance unit has been formed to provide a speedy and efficient service using either scheduled airline flights or specially prepared air ambulances. St John's co-operate with the Automobile Association air ambulance service.

It was in 1909 that the title Aerial Association was registered. Flying was still in its infancy and the idea of the Automobile Association having its own aircraft met with opposition from sceptics. When the A.A. finally took to the skies in 1921, it was for traffic management for that year's Derby.

Until World War II they only provided general information,

traffic control and weather reports for owners of light aircraft and during the war their flying activites ceased, all A.A. equipment being handed to the Air Ministry. It was not until 17 years later that the Association was again airborne. Their aircraft were up-dated regularly to meet the changing requirements of the A.A.; low level flying for map preparation and photographic work; however, the need for an air ambulance service became apparent.

It was largely with mercy missions in mind that the Association purchased a Cessna Golden Eagle in 1974. Four on-board computers, weather radar and automatic navigation systems made it one of the best and most comprehensively equipped small aircraft in the country at the time, but with room for only one stretcher case on board and with a range of 1,700 miles, the aircraft had its limitations.

Two Cessna 441 Conquests were bought in the early 80s and are the latest up-to-date machines. Their key roles are as air ambulances, flying sick and injured motorists home from the Continent. The accommodation is flexible for two stretcher cases with two trained attendants or 8 seated passengers.

These aircraft also participate in other roles - police liaison work, traffic control, photographic work, etc. They have a range of over 2,000 miles and a cruising speed of 330 miles per hour. The new Conquests more than adequately fulfill the Association's present needs and, with their increased capacity, range and speed, look set to cope with the ever-increasing demands of the later 80s. The following specification of the Cessna 441 'Conquest' should be compared with those used by the R.A.F. 60-odd years ago -

Fully equipped with the latest communication units and some medical appliances.

Engine   Twin engines. Garrett Air Research. Type 331-8-401S units. Turbo prop.Flat rated 625 SHP to 16,000 ft (4877 m).

Maximum speed	547 km/hr (295 knots) @ 16,000 ft
Cruising speed	543 km/hr (293 knots) @ 24,000 ft
Range (fuel)	2,070 n.miles + 45 minutes reserve
Accommodation	2 stretchers or 8 passengers
Crew	Pilot, Attendant
Dimensions	
Wingspan	150.57 m (592.8 inches)
Length	118.87 m (468 inches)
Height	39.93 m (157.2 inches)
Gross weight	4501.1 Kg (9925 lb)

Special features   VHF radio for air/ground communication with A.A.network; dual VHF transceivers; single UHF; single HF; dual VOR; dual ADF; dual DME; dual weather radar; integrated flight director system interlinked to auto-pilot.

Ambulance Trains

The usual question is asked. When were hospital trains first used? From the invention of Stephenson's steam engine and the inauguration of the first railway in England, tracks were quickly laid in many countries and it became obvious that here was a system to take troops quickly to the frontiers of those countries in the event of a threat of conflict. However, if troops could be carried a great distance by railway to make combat, then why not casualties resulting be taken by rail on the train's return journey?

It is not really certain when the railways were first used for medical duties; the earliest recorded occasion was the Crimean War in 1854, when wagons ran on a special track being constructed to take supplies to the front line. These wagons were supplying the troops and returning with the sick and wounded soldiers to the first aid posts. At first, the wagons were drawn by horses, followed later, as the track extended, by the use of a stationary steam engine assisting the horse up the slopes. This power system was eventually replaced by steam locomotives.

Following this war, serious consideration was given to the conveyance of the wounded by the new railway systems, but, again, only during a war, this time by the Prussians. Up to 1860 the majority of patients travelled in wagons with only a covering of straw on the floor to lie on, but that year improvements were made and seriously wounded casualties were carried in stretchers suspended by support straps probably from the sides of the wagon; the less serious cases continued to be carried inside passenger coaches. Later, sacks filled with straw converted into stretchers to provide more comfort were tried.

The International Congress of the Red Cross Societies in 1869 resulted in the Prussian Government adopting a system used in the Franco-Prussian War of 1870. They had a good service for carrying the casualties by rail. The coaches were split up into grades of casualty: a set of coaches for the lying down patients; a set for the sitting cases. Personnel responsible were given their own coaches, other coaches were used for supplies, water, fuel, baggage, etc. However, despite the higher standard, discomfort still existed due to the time taken to travel to the field hospitals, sometimes as long as 8 days.

During the same period, Surgeon-General Sir T Longmore was considering a design for a conveyance on the railway to provide comfort for casualties. The result was a carriage constructed at the Metropolitan works in Birmingham. The function of the carriage was to transport patients by railway from Portsmouth to Netley Hospital. The accommodation was 8 bunks, 4 a side on which patients on stretchers could be placed. There was a heater stove, water closet flushed by water from a tank in the carriage roof and a sink. An 'attendant's seat was provided, under which there were lockers for medicines and other supplies, also hinged seats for the use of medical orderlies. To provide easy access, there was a side entrance as well as folding doors at each end. It appears that the design was very successful, as more ambulance carriages were built in 1885 and 1886.

During the South African War of 1899-1902 trains were specially converted for the movement of the sick and wounded British troops. It was then that the British Red Cross Society began its long and valued association with the Army Medical Authorities in the provisioning, equipping and operation of these special ambulance trains.

One ambulance train was prepared in Natal and was ready at the beginning of the War, another soon afterwards, whilst a further two came later from Cape Town. The ambulance trains were equipped, well fitted and adequately staffed, chiefly for the conveyance of stretcher or 'lying down' cases. The others were just improvised trains from first class corridor coaches without any major alterations and took the sitting cases and the convalescent patients, with no permanent staff; medical attention was given during journeys. A kitchen coach was available in 3 compartments, one part was the actual kitchen, one a pharmacy that could also have bunks for a small number of the staff, and the third was staff quarters to house the rest of the staff in bunks.

The first fully-equipped hospital train to be built in England was the result of an offer by H.R.H. Princess Christian of Schleswig-Holstein to the Red Cross Committee to fund such a train, which was designed by Sir John Furley, founder of the ambulance section of the Order of St John, in 1899 and named the "Princess Christian Hospital Train"; all funding was by donation, including that of the Princess herself.

Between the wars, 1902 to 1914, there was no demand for ambulance trains - normal home casualties had to make the best of it, with no public ambulance service available.

It was not until the Great War that the hospital train, renamed the 'ambulance train', came back into operation. No properly converted or constructed train was available in England to ship to France with the British Expeditionary Force. The intention was for the French railways to provide transport for the wounded to the French ports where the casualties would be transferred to hospital ships.

From 14th August, 1914, six detachments of the Royal Army Medical Corps, with 2 officers and 45 non-commissioned officers and men to each, were trained at Aldershot. Later all six were sent to Southampton: each was ready to man an ambulance train of 500 to 600 casualties. Eventually, they were shipped across the Channel to Boulogne, but without any trains to accompany them. The reason given was that, due to circumstances, it was impossible to ship even one ambulance train from England, but, worse still, there was not a single train ready. It was obvious that ambulance trains would have to be constructed from rolling stock obtained from the French railways.

There was no immediate problem for the sitting cases, who could usually be housed in the supply trains on their empty return to base. The serious difficulty was how to transport the stretcher or 'lying down' cases.

The first ambulance trains were made from French rolling stock; carriages, vans, and covered and open trucks. The conversion was reasonably easy for the carriages and the covered trucks – removing the seats from the carriages, scrubbing out all the vehicles and disinfecting them. Then came the problem of how to support stretchers to make beds. It must be remembered that at this period there were no motor ambulances available for the use of the R.A.M.C. in France. However, the British War Office had foreseen difficulties of this nature and had experimented with various stretcher supports. Finally, after much research, they had selected an iron stretcher carry apparatus, the "Bréchot-Déspres-Amelines", which could be installed in empty carriages or wagons. This was a contraption consisting of a length of angle iron formed into a loop representing an inverted letter 'U'. At each end of the upright was formed a foot to enable the support legs to be bolted to the floor. Connecting rods, 3 in all, were fixed across the open legs for rigidity. 3 formed rods were anchored in the proximity of the connecting rods, by coil tension springs, supporting the stretchers. Each upright was placed at a distance of 6 feet apart, loop uppermost and horizontal tie rods were attached to each upright to form a rigid structure. The whole apparatus was finally fixed to the floor. It would bear the weight of 3 casualties, each being well clear of the other patients. When not in use the apparatus was unscrewed from the floor, the ties removed and the whole structure stacked with others at the end of the carriage or wagon.

Amiens was the Base of the British Army and the Medical Corps. It was not possible to convert any railway stock immediately at the start of the War, even had the vehicles been available, to

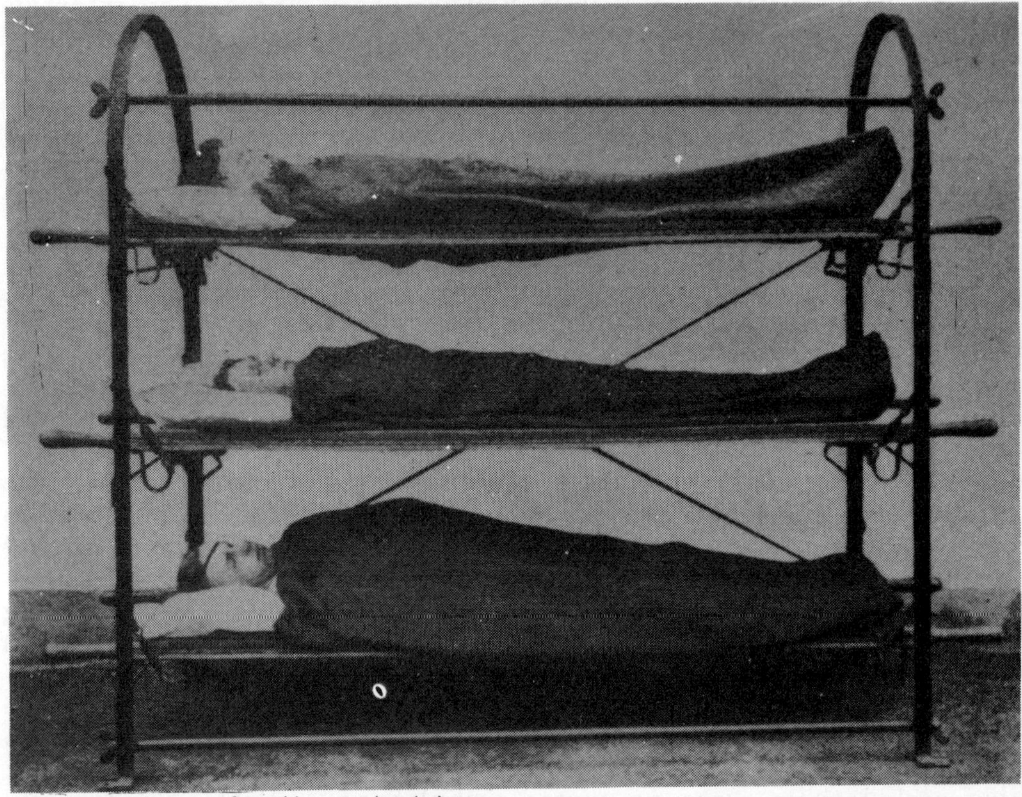

The Brechot carrying three stretchers

place on the track as the French railways were taxed to the hilt in conveying troops, food and munitions to the front. It was not until 17th August at a large junction a mile from Amiens that there was any activity on ambulance trains, when wagons, a few carriages and luggage vans became available and were handed over to the British.

This was the beginning of the British Ambulance Train Service.

300 men of the Royal Army Medical Corps worked night and day to convert this rolling stock into some semblance of ambulance trains. They first divided the rolling stock into three train sets. After clearing and cleaning, sets of "Brechot apparatus" were fitted in the empty wagons, 4 to each, providing transport for 12 stretcher casualties per wagon. Well equipped wards, surgical dressing areas, stores equipment and food, blankets, etc. were provided. The one important thing about these heavy wagons was the hard suspension; with only the weight of 12 men the springs did not even deflect, never mind operate, they stayed as solid beams, which was uncomfortable for the wounded. Of the other rolling stock, some carriages were converted into kitchens with their chimneys poking through holes in their roofs, each kitchen being capable of catering for about 700 patients. Barrels of fresh water were

installed, also filters, ice chests and disinfecting apparatus.

Here were the first three ambulance trains. Meanwhile, difficulty was being experienced in obtaining the medical supplies, reserve blankets and stretchers, pails, jugs, basins, etc. - essential items for the requirements of 700 patients! Unfortunately, these articles could not be supplied by the Royal Army Ordnance Department. However, a high-ranking officer granted permission for the necessary supplies to be purchased locally, debiting the account to the British Government. This was a step in the right direction to ensure the success of the three trains. Each Train Commander scoured the shops in the town bringing back to the depot the required stores for their trains. To get the articles not obtainable in Amiens, one Commander left for Paris with the purchasing authority to buy the outstanding stores and equipment.

During the time the ambulance trains were under construction, medical aid was provided by the food supply trains leaving daily for the front line. In each of these trains one of the vans was equipped with 12 folding "Brechot apparatus" to carry 36 'lying down' and 80 sitting casualties, and with medical stores and equipment for taking the wounded on the return journey to the base. On arrival, the vans were unloaded, scrubbed and disinfected before the supply train started on its next journey to the front line.

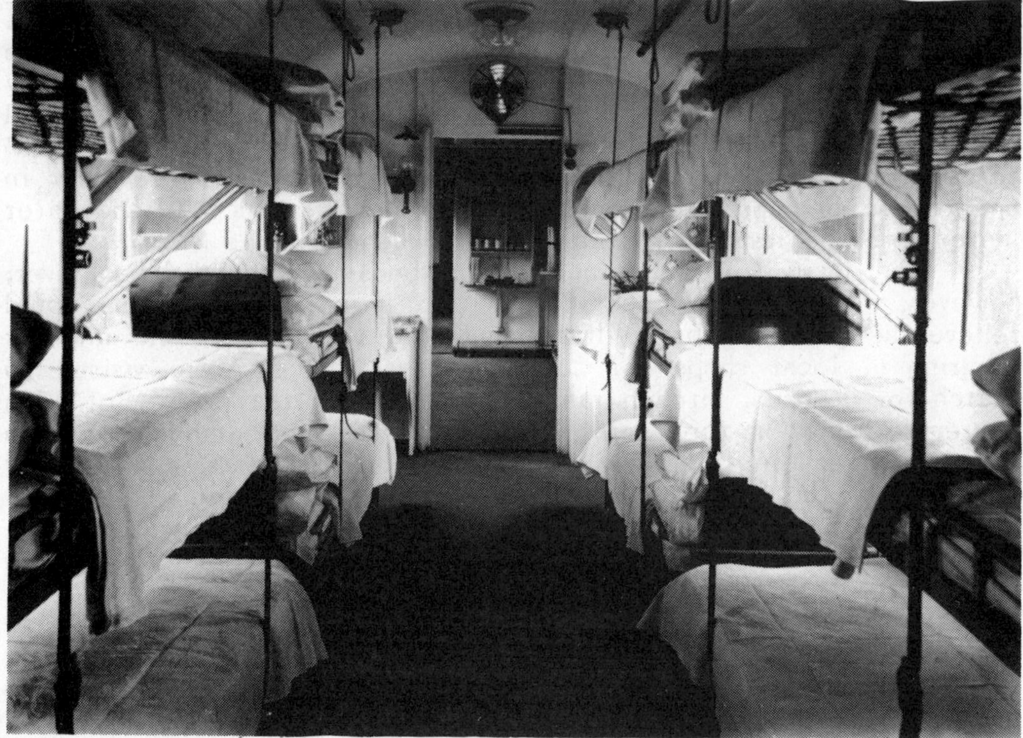

L.Y.R. ambulance train (interior of ward and pharmacy for serious cases), 1914-18 (by permission of the National Railway Museum)

The work on the ambulance trains continued until 26th August when, as complete as possible, they steamed out on their first trips to the fighting front line. The next job was to convert further trains, which were made up of 3rd class carriages from which the seats had been removed. On 27th August, No. 4 and 5 personnel were transferred to Rouen because of the German advance on Amiens. On 30th August No. 4 was completed and began its duties.

If more trains were to be converted further rolling stock was required. Every effort was made by approaching everyone in authority for assistance in providing more rolling stock. At last the French Government was asked for help but, due to the retreat from Mons, great pressure had been put on to the French Army with a tremendous need for transport for the sick and wounded, which made their needs greater than the British, so any idea of even borrowing a train became impossible.

The situation at Rouen was getting worse as the enemy advanced rapidly. However, the situation improved when a French ambulance train arrived on the scene. The British approached the French Commandant about the British wounded and their urgent need of ambulance train transport for casualties in the fighting around Paris. The result was a merger of British and French, whereby 45 R.A.M.C. personnel, with stores and equipment, joined the French train with its own staff of officers and 25 men. At 1 a.m. on 31st August, the combined British and French train, "Entente Cordiale", moved off for Attiche; renamed "Franco-British" by September it had almost become a hospital train. Carriages had been partitioned off as wards for various surgical and medical cases; storerooms, offices and well-equipped kitchens were fully in operation. This combined ambulance train was a success and later moved into the ranks with the others to be known as No. 6.

The need for ambulance trains became greater than ever; however, at Villeneuve, near Paris, two more French trains could relieve the situation, but still needing converting. There was another scouring of local shops for supplies, other places were visited to search for utensils, kitchen ranges, etc., and on the evening of 15th September one of the trains was completed and ambulance train No. 5 left for the front. Two days later the second train was ready and left for the forward area as No. 7 ambulance train.

This latter was the first to be caught by enemy action at the height of the Battle of Ypres. The train was badly damaged but, worst of all, it was immobile as the engine had gone in search of water. Eventually it was moved and delivered the wounded to base station in spite of its damaged condition.

By 20th September, 1914, the British had 7 ambulance trains operating continually and achieving remarkable results. As more troops arrived from England, so the casualties mounted and more ambulance trains were needed. From where? That was the great question. Three more French trains were applied for, but were never forthcoming; efforts were also made to obtain any carriages at Villeneuve to replace the original heavy rolling stock used for ambulance trains No.s 1, 2 and 3.

Nursing sisters were now carrying out regular duties on the ambulance trains. For every train there was a Commander whose duties were to estimate quantities of supplies, food and medical stores required, get them, and have the train prepared ready for action.

On 21st September, a Red Cross Society Ambulance Train appeared and a few hours later, a second. These trains were small, taking only 200 cases each, so to provide a more suitable unit the trains were joined together. The staff was increased and, the next day the ambulance train set off on its errand of mercy. Even with the increased capacity through the merger, it was not really sufficient and after only one journey the rolling stock was integrated into other trains.

At this time a party was at Villeneuve collecting carriages to form another improvised ambulance train, No. 8, which started on its first trip on 3rd October. 30th October saw a further train, No. 9, on its maiden voyage; it consisted of a number of luggage vans converted into well heated and comfortable wards.

The next, No. 10, companion to No. 9, followed on 9th November. The Red Cross Society and the St John Ambulance Association began to convert French first class cariages at Sotterville. The whole of this latest train featured ideas by Sir John Furley, who helped with its construction. The fittings were made in England by the Birmingham Carriage and Railway Wagon Company and shipped to France for this particular train. However, whilst it improved the comfort of the casualties by the installation of Furley's stretcher-beds, it had no connecting passages between the carriages and therefore each ward was almost self-contained and supported by its own staff. Designated as No. 11, it steamed out on its initial journey on 9th November.

Stationed near the ambulance station and train factory at Boulogne was a small group of women who had established themselves as an organisation later to become one of the most successful groups of the War. This was the Voluntary Aid Detachment (V.A.D.) of the British Red Cross, which had been inaugurated in England some years earlier. Their members had all been trained in all aspects of hospital work and organisation, as compounders, cooks, clerks, quartermasters, store keepers and all were certificated in first aid and nursing duties. At first the group assisted at Boulogne in handling the large number of wounded arriving there continuously, but later they were given the task of looking after the hosts of invalids and other troops passing the station at a rate of hundreds a day.

A properly fitted, equipped and furnished ambulance train, made up from some of the Home Units arrived from England - Train No. 12. All the heavy wagons and vans which had been initially converted into ambulance trains, Nos. 1, 2 and 3, were replaced by first and second class coaches converted to carry the various classes of wounded and sick. To get the best comfort for the casualties, the first class accommodation for the serious stretcher cases were well sprung. The seats had been widened in some coaches to enable patients in a less serious condition to lie down in reasonable comfort. Such cases as skin infection, mental problems, and other types of infectious cases who were able to sit up and feed themselves were accommodated in the converted second class carriages. Two kitchens were provided in each train, one located near the end of the train and the other in the middle, which facilitated cooking for the different classes of patient.

The next arrival from England was No. 14 (No. 13 had been omitted), donated by the Lord and Lady Michelham and christened "Queen Mary's Ambulance Train". Further ambulance trains appeared, Nos. 15, 16, 17 and 18 and, later, Nos. 21, 22, and 24. No. 15 was donated by Princess Christian.

Ten coaches were built by the Birmingham Carriage and Railway Wagon Company, as was the one sent to South Africa, which was specially constructed for the purpose of a hospital train. Nos. 16 and 17, two more specially built ambulance trains provided by the United Kingdom Flour Millers' Association, were approved by the War Office and included the latest developments in ambulance train transport.

In 1916 ten more ambulance trains appeared in France - these were Nos. 19, 20, 23, 25 to 31 (inclusive). The ambulance trains 26 to 38 were of a standard pattern produced in line with specifications set by the Ambulance Train Committee. This Committee was inaugurated in France to review the reports and suggestions of the medical officers in charge of train units during the first years of the war. Nos. 39, 41, 42 and 43 were still being built to the same pattern with increased accommodation. Ambulance trains 42 and 43 reached their destination in 1918.

Throughout the war the British Ambulance Train Service in France did a remarkable job. 3,400,000 sick and wounded were brought from the front to base medical stations or hospitals, with 1,600,000 carried between bases, totalling over 5 million conveyed to receive treatment between August, 1914 and November, 1918.

There were a number of ambulance trains in Britain; the various railway companies initially had 12 ambulances. At the start of the war Southampton became a military port where casualties were taken from the arriving hospital ships. Some patients were taken from Southampton by the ambulance trains to the Royal Victoria Hospital at Netley, and some to Well Hall in Kent.

The staff of the hospital ships labelled the patients with their area destination, such as London and Southern, West of England, North England, Scotland or Ireland. The area chosen was the nearest to the patient's home town, where he could be sent to a local hospital. Large hospitals sent their patients, when fit to travel, to smaller military, civilian and private hospitals and convalescent homes as near to the patient's home as possible. This left more beds vacant for incoming sick and wounded from the ambulance trains. From the original 12 the service grew to 372 ambulance trains by April, 1918, the trains operating at the average of 12 per day.

To give an indication of the size of the problem – one battle, that of the Somme, in 1916, produced 68,000 casualties reaching Southampton and 49,000 arriving at Dover: 117,000 in all.

The Navy had their own ambulance train service within the United Kingdom during the Great War. Whilst it is not intended to detail the operation of this service, it can be said that it was very similar to that of the military ambulance train service at home. The main difference was in the type of cots or beds used by the Navy, who preferred moveable cots instead of the military fixed type. The reason was that casualties could be placed in a medical cot in the ship in which they were serving or in the Naval Hospital Ship and could then be carried in the cot to an ambulance train remaining undisturbed. It saved the transfer of a patient from cot to stretcher, then back to cot or bed on the train, and then to bed in the hospital. Objections to the army fixed cot was that it was subjected to every movement of the ambulance coach when the train was in motion, while the Navel moveable cot reduced this movement to a minimum.

Information about ambulance trains during World War II is not as detailed or as readily available as it was for the Great War. This is probably due to the improvisation of Frencn trains which virtually started the ambulance train service in 1914. Since then experience had been gained and a great deal of preparation carried out by 1939. Prior to war being declared much thought had been given by the British Government to the safety of the civilian population, as well as the troops. Work on the railways, such as building new rolling stock and steam locomotives, had ceased by official order and the railway workshops were being equipped for the manufacture of tanks, guns and other heavy type munitions. It was in mid-1939 when the Government decided it was necessary to have a number of ambulance trains prepared for the evacuation of the people injured during the anticipated air attacks on Britain or during a possible invasion.

It was thought that something like 34 trains would be

needed, each with 10 corridor vans and 2 brake vans, converted to take stretcher cases. The railway companies were not in agreement as these corridor vans were required to operate within their normal traffic and, as no replacements would be forthcoming, they could not be released. However, the companies did agree that the rolling stock would be made available to the Government when the emergency arose. To ensure that the vans could be quickly adapted, special brackets were produced to support the stretchers and stored in boxes on the underframe of the vans. The brake vans were fitted out with shelves and cupboards for medical stores, ready for ambulance operation when necessary.

Just before the war began the railway companies had consulted the War Office with plans to convert the first 12 trains; 8 for the Home Front and 4 for European operation. Each ambulance train would consist of 9 carriages of 7 different types (some time later two more pieces of rolling stock were added). At home conversion was for resident doctors; nurses; stretcher patients' ward; sitting patients' ward; special part for mental cases; kitchen car; and space for medical supplies and other stores. For overseas duties the ambulance train had 16 carriages and vans, 9 different types, and provided with steam couplings and draw-gear suitable for continental use, to be connected to French locomotives.

On 2nd September, 1939, Government instructions to the railway companies were to proceed with the actual conversions of the first 12 trains. The carriages, vans and necessary equipment were sent to the workshops of the 4 companies to make the conversions and equipment installations. After some three weeks two complete ambulance trains were ready for the Home Front and four specially equipped for overseas operation, all being handed over to the military command.

By the end of the first quarter of 1940, 25 trains had been converted and prepared for duty, 12 at home and 13 for overseas, involving 344 carriages and wagons from the London, Midland & Scottish Railway. Unfortunately, 9 of those shipped overseas to France were lost. It should be noted that during the evacuation of the B.E.F. and other troops from Dunkirk and other French ports from the end of May to 10th June, 1940, the casualties carried in 47 ambulance trains were approximately 31,000, subsequently admitted to military and civilian hospitals in the United Kingdom.

By August, 1942, 23 more trains were required for overseas by the Allied Forces. It was decided to reduce the number of ward coaches, so the trains were reduced by two. A further decision was that each railway should convert its own rolling stock.

More orders increased the number of ambulances to 66. At this time, the number of coaches, corridor vans, wagons and brake vans involved in the conversions was 925. The distribution among the railways workshops was Swindon 154; Derby and Wolverton 343;

Doncaster and York 290; Eastleigh and Lancing 138.

The American Forces in the United Kingdom also needed a number of ambulance trains. The first of these was converted from the rolling stock of the Great Western, completed and handed over to the American Command on 25th March, 1943. G.W.R. constructed a siding specially at Shrivenham, Wiltshire, to receive American casualties.

By 'D-Day' (6th June, 1944) there were 32 ambulance trains for the British Army and 34 for American forces. American casualties brought back from Normandy were distributed to the hospitals using 5 of the British trains and 10 American. These trains were awaiting shipment to the continent later. London & North Eastern Railway locomotives, fitted with Westinghouse vacuum braking system, were used exclusively as these were considered the only available locomotives suitable to couple to the American type ambulance rolling stock fitted with the same braking system.

From the first ambulance train journey at the start of operations just after 'D-Day' to 8th May, 1945, over 1,800 journeys were made with a full complement of staff within Great Britain, carrying 360,000 casualties.

The programme of evacuation of casualties in this country was developed using 34 ambulance trains, which were mainly used for clearing the population from danger areas, taking the sick and wounded from ports to hospitals supplementing the Army ambulance trains, and for transferring large number of casualties from one area to another. In the end these evacuation trains were little used for their main intention to move air raid casualties.

To complete the Second World War record the total number of casualties carried from 'D-Day' to the date when the evacuation train service ceased was 192,551 – including 152,492 service personnel, made up by 101,900 British, 47,319 American and 3,273 Canadians.

This is not all the story of the ambulance trains and certainly not the end, for after the war they continued to function with the British Army of the Rhine (B.A.O.R.). 33 German railway carriages had been converted into ambulance trains and 11 were allocated to each train. There were the usual staff cars, kitchens, wards, pharmacy coach, etc. These three trains were used to take patients from Trieste and Austria to B.A.O.R. until 1964, when the trains were taken over by the Royal Corps of Transport. The conversion and installations were pretty well similar to the coaches of the older type during the two world wars.

What of the future? It is anticipated that the military ambulance train will for the time being be similar to the standard design used in the past. Equipment will be improved, with the latest in medical care, and with better catering facilities. As for civilian requirements, any long distance journeys made for medical reasons can be made with the help of the British Railways Board.

Travelling by rail, in addition to being more economical than ambulance transport in most cases, can ensure greater comfort for the patients travelling long distances. The use of rail transport should be considered and is dependent upon medical advice for each individual case.

There is no special accommodation available and, with the design of coaches now in use, it is not usually possible to take stretcher cases by rail. However, the use of sleeping car trains may sometimes be practicable and special facilities are also available for people travelling with wheelchairs by train.

The railway authorities will always assist and make recommendations for the use of available services. There is co-operation between the railways and the ambulance services for carriage between the railway stations and hospitals.

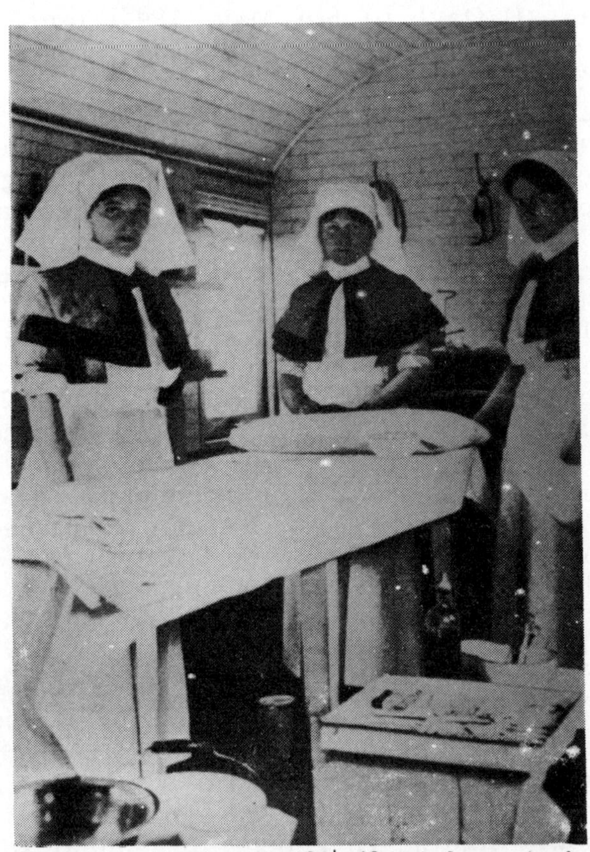

Operating theatre on 1914-18 ambulance train

Hospital Ships

The two ambulance services that worked closely together during the four conflicts from 1854 to 1945 were the ambulance train service and the hospital ship organisation.

When did the hospital and/or ambulance ship really start in service? Records give dates of some operating during the 16th century, when it was possible that the Spanish Armada, as well equipped and organised as history would suggest, certainly would have facilities to look after the seriously wounded officers and men – or just officers!

Britain's first recorded ship set aside for hospital duties was the 'Goodwill' in 1608. Although two more such ships sailed with a West Indies expedition in 1654, it was not until after the Restoration in 1660 that the Royal Navy made a point of ensuring that certain ships would be made available when required for such a purpose. Some of the earlier ships would have been appropriately called ambulance ships for the taking of serious sea casualties to ports where further transport took them to hospitals or lodging houses on shore.

When a fleet of 29 English ships, including 9 warships, sailed in 1683 to assist in the evacuation of Tangier, two of the naval ships, the 'Unity' and the 'Welcome' were fitted out as hospital ships.

Ships commissioned for hospital work during the 18th century had a number of personnel responsible, 5 nurses and 3 launderesses in addition to 8 assistants in each ship. Fighting ships no longer required or suitable for active service were permanently converted to hospital ships. Gun decks were cleared, cabins and bulkheads removed, and to separate the classes of casualties canvas partitions were erected to separate wards.

As time went by and medical progress was made, these special ships became larger and equipped for full medical attention and some had areas set aside where surgery could be carried out, after which the patient could convalesce until fit to re-join his own ship. These vessels could rightly be termed hospital ships. Some did take to port and anchor near to do a period of duty as floating base hospitals.

Britain was the greatest user of such ships, which were part of the Royal Navy, dealing with the casualties during and after sea battles, performing operations for the survival of the men. These ships still did their duty during peacetime, looking after the sick as part of the fleets at sea. These worthy vessels received the honour of being designated H.M.H.S. (His/Her Majesty's Hospital Ship).

Before separate ships were created to take care of the casualties transferred from the fighting ships, all vessels had a naval surgeon and a complement of men aboard, while some ships also had sick berth facilities.

In 1882 the P & O (Peninsular & Orient Steam Navigation Company) liner 'Carthage' served as a hospital ship on two voyages to Alexandria during the Arabi Pasha rebellion. During the 1883 campaign in the Sudan, the 'Ganges' was converted to a hospital ship, fitted out with different wards on different decks and with special accommodation for the mental and convalescent patients.

There were civilian hospital ships operating on African rivers and lakes, one of these being in connection with the expedition to the Sudan in 1898. Permission was obtained from Cairo to use river boats to transfer the casualties to hospitals by the Nile and save the long and fatiguing rail journey. A large, swift boat already on the river, called the 'Mayflower', was chartered and arrangements were made to convert her into a hospital ship to carry 52 patients, and in an emergency she could take a further 20 casualties. The ship was installed with the latest medical equipment and began her first voyage from Assuan on 15th September for Cairo where she put into port on 18th September. Her full complement was 4 officers and 27 other ranks, among the wounded were 2 officers and 17 men suffering from dysentary and fever. The 'Mayflower' continued to travel back and forth between Cairo and Assuan until mid-October.

In October, 1868, a Diplomatic Conference had been held in Geneva, where the first principles on maritime warfare were laid down. Other conferences were held on various points to be adopted. One held at the Hague to consider revisions relating to maritime warfare was completed in October, 1907, on certain conditions under which hospital ships were entitled to immunity from attack.

The Boer war saw many hospital ships, both Naval and Military, in action. Two ships, one launched in 1880, the 'Spartan', converted after being requisitioned at Southampton in 1899, the other her sister ship, the 'Trojan', launched in 1881, was also requisitioned and converted. The 'Spartan' carried the sick and wounded from Durban to Cape Town base hospital.

During the Great War a great many changes were made. Due to the considerable number of casualties starting to overcrowd the hospital ships available, they were unable to continue as real hospital ships either at sea or as base hospitals. They had to adopt

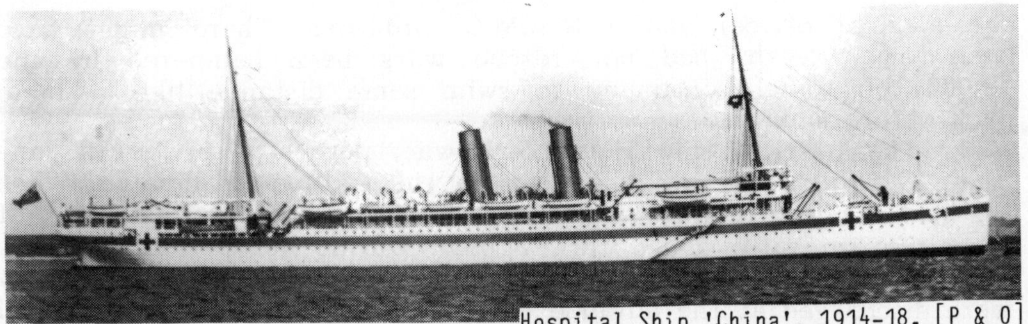

Hospital Ship 'China', 1914-18. [P & O]

the role of ambulance carriers, treating the casualties and then taking the serious cases to the shore based hospitals.

A large number of ships were mobilised to act as ambulances, supplying a more frequent service between the French ports and the home base hospitals. The P & O Group allocated some 28 of their ships for use as hospital ships or ambulance transports. Such vessels as the 'China', 'Devanha', 'Sicilia', 'Soudan', 'Syria', 'Madras' and 'Varsova' were on these duties throughout the war.

At the beginning of the war the Admiralty considered the requisitioning of ocean liners to convert them into hospital ships. Initially, 3 were commandeered and converted, accommodating between 200 and 300 beds each. Later they were joined by a further six. The British India Steam Navigation Company (B.I.) [later taken over by P & O] provided 2 ships, the 'Karapara' and the 'Vasna', which were converted into hospital ships, remaining as such.

Among the naval hospital ships serving during the conflict was the 'St Margaret of Scotland', equipped by the Scottish branch of the British Red Cross Society. The money raised for the funding of this ship also provided motor boats suitable as sea ambulances for operation in the Dardanelles, Egypt and Salonika. In the Battle of Jutland the collecting and transporting of casualties from the fighting ships to the hospital ships was carried out by this type of small ambulance motor boat.

From Scapa Flow to Gallipoli, East Africa to Mesopotamia, hospital and ambulance ships carried and cared for the wounded. There were casualties among the hospital ships themselves, which were certainly not free to operate despite the Geneva Convention. Of the P & O ships the 'Rohilla' was wrecked off Whitby in October, 1914. A military hospital ship on active service, the 'Britannic' was sunk by a mine at 8.12 a.m. on 21st November, 1916, in the Aegean Sea on her way to Mudros on the island of Limnos (Lemnos) off the east coast of Turkey. The weather was warm and the sea calm. No patients were on board, only the crew of 1,125 and medical staff of 25 medical officers, 76 nursing sisters and 399 R.A.M.C. and other ranks. There were 34 fatal casualties, including one medical officer and 8 R.A.M.C. orderlies. There might have been fewer deaths had not rescue work been hampered by the 48,000 ton vessel continuing to swim some distance like a lame duck before sinking.

The hospital ship H.M.H.S. 'Rewa', put into service in January, 1915, achieved great success in the Gallipoli campaign. When she had completed her assignment, she left with her last load of casualties in April, bound for England. During her period of operation as hospital ship she had taken 7,424 patients on board – 3,647 were discharged at the advance base, 3,628 had been taken to naval hospitals at Malta, Alexandria and Plymouth and 149 had died on board. Eventually, after three years, the good ship, though clearly marked as a hospital ship, was torpedoed in January, 1918, south-west of Lundy Island when approaching the Bristol Channel. Four of the engine room crew were killed; the explosion shattering two lifeboats, but two nearby ships picked up the casualties and the rest of the crew and took them to Swansea the following day.

In the summer of 1915, the British Red Cross commissioned two motor launches as river ambulance boats for Mesopotamia to evacuate casualties along the River Tigris.

The antagonists obeyed the Geneva Convention regarding hospital ships with reluctance. Hazards continued to face the white ships, whether military or naval. Between the years 1915 and 1917, seven military hospital ships struck mines and were either badly damaged, sunk or repaired.

In 1917, the Central Powers decided to disregard the International law, irrespective of the hospital ships being marked to distinguish them from members of the fighting forces; hospital ships would no longer be protected by the Geneva Convention. After this decision, the first British hospital ship to be torpedoed in 1917 was the 'Asturias' and in the next two years, a further 8 were to meet the same fate – the resulting casualties were very heavy indeed.

The 'Madras' was in Vladivostock in 1918; the 'Kalyan' supported the campaign in Northern Russia and was frozen in at Archangel on the White Sea over the winter of 1918-19. Hospital ships, 'Vasna' and 'Varela' were released from service in 1921.

When World War II came designs and development in the shipbuilding and engineering industries, leading to greater use of hospital ships equipped with the latest developments of medical science.

In the evacuation of Dunkirk many ships and boats of all sizes were engaged. Cross Channel steamers owned by the railway companies were brought into action, many of them being converted into hospital ships or ambulance carriers. One of these steamers, the 'Brighton', carried out a regular trip between Dieppe and Newhaven and had, at times, as many as 250 casualties aboard. Unfortunately she was sunk in an air raid. Another Cross Channel steamer owned by the Southern Railway already converted, the 'Maid of Kent' bearing the appropriate markings and the Red Cross, was bombed and sunk at Dieppe. Ten railway steamships were converted into hospital ships and ambulances for the British Expeditionary Force. During the evacuation this small fleet of ships carried more than 20,000 casualties to British ports.

P & O's contribution was by one of their groups, the B I, to the hospital ship fleet; the 'Karapara', the 'Vasna' and the 'Vita' had all seen service in the first war and four more converted liners joined their ranks. They were to be found off Abyssinia and Somaliland, off Libya and in the South Atlantic. The 'Talamba' brought back the survivors from the battleships 'Prince of Wales' and 'Repulse' and 'Vita' survivors from H.M.S.'Hermes'. These ships went to Diego Suarez, north of Madagascar. Four followed the fleet to the invasion of Sicily, during which campaign the 'Talamba' was sunk. The 'Vita' and the 'Vasna' went to Burma and the 'Vasna' ended her war career repatriating invalid prisoners-of-war from Japan. Another ship, the 'Llandovery Castle', the successor to its namesake which was sunk in the Great War, went to Tobruk after the victory at El Alamein, arriving in November, 1942, to pick up

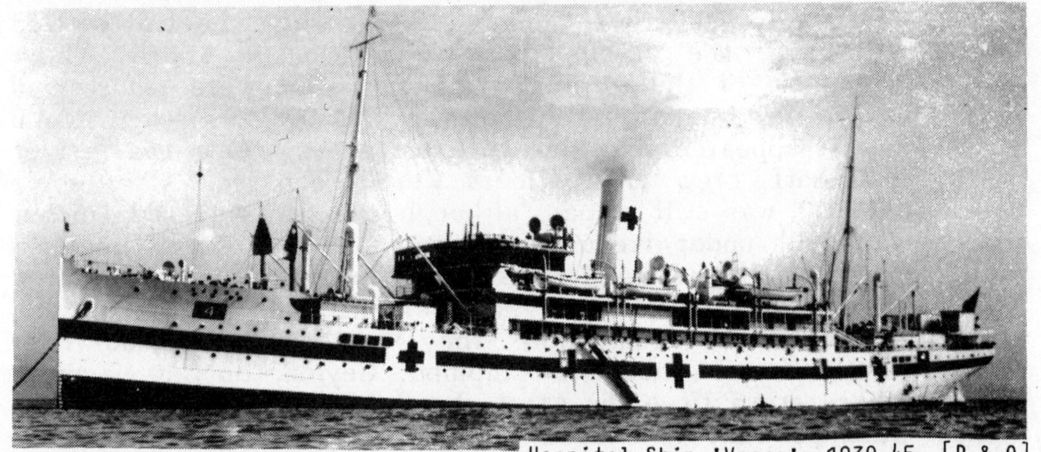

Hospital Ship 'Vasna', 1939-45. [P & O]

715 casualties and take them to Alexandria. A number of hospital ships which had already been involved in major operations at Dunkirk, served in the Mediterranean between 1943 and 1944, taking casualties from the beaches during landing operations, while keeping close to the coast line as possible. To help casualties from the beaches, lifeboats called 'water ambulances' equipped to carry stretcher cases, were sent out from the hospital ships. These 'Water ambulances' were made of light material and with flat bottoms were able to negociate part way up the beaches. Two hospital ships, the 'St Andrew' and the 'St David' arrived in the Mediterranean in June, 1943, for the landings at Salerno, Italy, on the coast of the Tyrrhenian Sea. Air attacks against them were

frequent and eventually the 'St David' was hit and sank 25 miles from Anzio in January, 1944: 55 lives were lost, including the captain of the ship, the commanding officer, a medical officer and two nurses. Her sister ship had carried 6,000 patients, travelling some 25,000 miles: she made 37 trips to Anzio, carrying casualties from Ancona to Bari, both on the Adriatic Coast of Italy. Later, in September, 1944, on her last voyage between Ancona and Bari, she struck a mine; luckily her damage was not too great, as she was able to be towed into Taranto in the heel of Italy and later brought home to Birkenhead for repair.

There is a story of one hospital ship with a great adventure. The 'Vita' was requisitioned in May, 1940, and was converted into a hospital ship in Bombay that August, her first voyage being from Berbera in Somalia. For 6 months the 'Vita' was the base hospital in Aden. She travelled to Tobruk where, lying off the coast loaded with some 400 patients, she was attacked by enemy aircraft, fortunately without being hit. However, one near miss did a lot of damage to her superstructure when the blast lifted her stern completely out of the sea. That was not the only damage, the engines and the dynamos were put out of action, five wards were wrecked and there was other damage. Later, when she had settled down in the sea, she developed a serious list to port. Whilst patients and some of the medical staff and crew were transferred to H.M.H.S.'Waterhen', others of the staff and officers remained on board. When it appeared that she would go at any time, the rest of the medical staff, crew and officers were evacuated. After some time, the 'Vita' was still afloat, although she had suffered further air attacks. Still under frequent attack, she was towed to Port Said, through the Suez Canal, to Tewfik, stopping there for repairs. Afterwards she was rejoined by her own medical staff and crew and returned to Aden. From there, the 'Vita' went to Addu Attol in 1941 and then continued to Colombo, Ceylon, on 1st January, 1942. On her return to Addu Attol she found the survivors of two British warships that had been sunk by Japanese aircraft. The 'Vita' rescued 595 survivors, during which time the Japanese honoured the status of the hospital ship and any further air attacks ceased. Six days later, again in Addu Attol, further casualties were rescued and taken to Durban.

After some time at Kilindini, she went to Bombay for a refit, leaving there when completed in September for hospital duty at Diego Suarez. She continued with her duties with the Eastern Fleet in the beginning of 1944 and then again returned to Bombay. At Trincomalee the 'Vita' had a spell of base hospital duty. This did not last long, as she was instructed to act as a hospital carrier between Colombo and Durban, finishing at Cochin in southern India in April, 1945. Further travels then took the 'Vita' to collect casualties from Rangoon and take them to Calcutta. During the retreat of the Japanese from Burma she made a voyage to Chittagong, where casualties were taken aboard and went to Madras. Back again to Trincomalee as a base hospital, afterwards making her last voyage to Bombay for another refit. The 'Vita's ' busy and adventurous life as hospital ship, carrier and base hospital ended at the beginning of 1946 when she was paid off.

During the war about 50 motor fishing vessels were equipped with medical supplies and adapted to carry 8 to 10 stretchers of beds and from 12 to 20 sitting and mobile patients. These boats were used alongside hospital carriers and other ships which were anchored outside ports and harbours. Their function was to unload casualties from the ships and bring them ashore to the base hospitals and to take invalids from one port or harbour to another along the coast. Some of these M.F.V.s were used during the North African operations and the Italian campaign, and in Indian and Ceylonese ports. Four were attached to the British Pacific Fleet in 1944, carrying out their duties at Sydney, Brisbane and Freemantle.

After the World war shipping reverted to its civilian role, but it was always there ready for any further action they might be asked to support.

During the Korean campaign H.M.H.S. 'Maine' was used extensively for ferrying U.N. casualties from Korea to the United States Army base hospitals in Japan. Accommodation in the 'Maine' at that time was two decks of wards, upper level 116 double tiered beds and divided into 5 wards; the lower level 156 double-tiered beds, also divided into 5 wards. There were medical and surgical facilities, an X-ray department, and a dispensary. The 'Maine' came from a long line of hospital ships bearing her name. The first began as a base military hospital ship in 1900, but ran ashore in thick fog and was abandoned. The line continued until the last one was commissioned in 1950, placed at the disposal of the United Nations and sent to Korea. H.M.H.S. 'Maine' ended her service on 26th April, 1954, in Hong Kong where she was sold and broken up.

On 9th April, 1982, two of P & O's liners, the 'Canberra' and the 'Elk' left with the task force for the Falkland Islands. Several other ships joined the fleet, including the 'Strathewe', 'Norland' and 'Uganda'. Whilst the 'Canberra' did perform as a hospital ship, her principle function was that of a troop carrier. The real hospital ship was the 'Uganda', the others were really for the conveyance of troops, equipment and supplies.

The 'Uganda' had a crew of 271 and 40 nurses of the Queen Alexandra's Royal Nursing Service, the first time that female nurses had been to sea since the Korean War. All her public rooms were converted to set up the hospital facilities which included an operating theatre, burns units wards, X-ray failities, a dental surgery and an opthalmology department. Even the ship's cocktail bar was converted into a pathology laboratory.

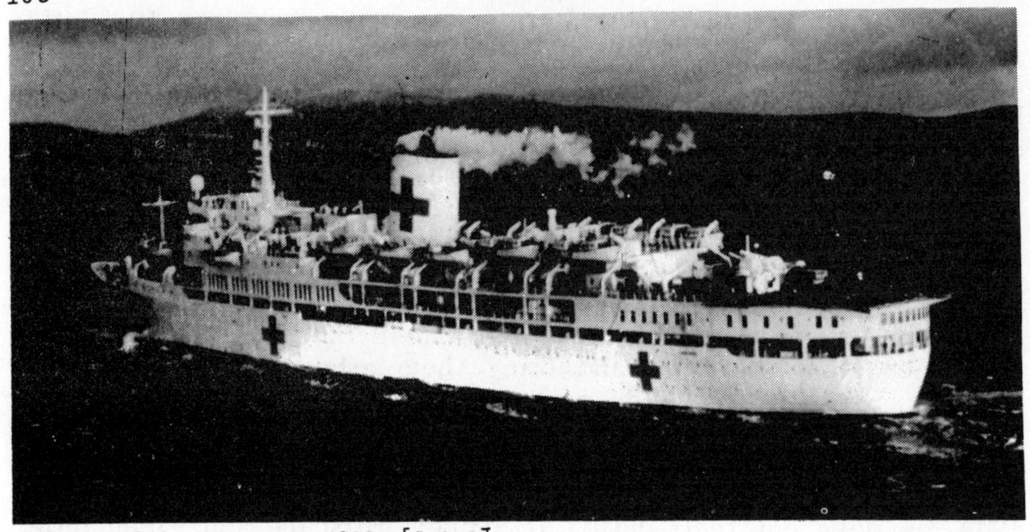

Hospital Ship 'Uganda', 1982. [P & O]

The first casualties were from the guided missile destroyer, H.M.S.'Sheffield', who arrived on 12th May: the last casualties were taken aboard at Port Stanley on 13th July. She treated a total of 730 casualties, 150 of them Argentinian prisoners, with the ship's surgeons carrying out some 500 operations. The 'Uganda' operated in conjunction with three ambulance ships, the 'Hecla', the 'Hydra' and the 'Herald', survey vessels converted to ferry casualties from the 'Uganda' to the Uruguyan capital of Montevideo, thence to be flown back to Britain by the R.A.F.

The 'Uganda' was at one stage co-ordinating the movements of three Argentinian hospital ships, the 'Bahia Paraise', the 'Almirante Inzar' and the 'Puerto Deseado', as well as those of four other British hospital and ambulance ships. She returned home the 'heroine' of the hour. She was de-registered as a hospital ship on 13th July, when the Red Crosses were painted out. Following an extensive refit in Tyneside, she was scheduled to resume her normal cruising on 25th September with a 14 night cruise to the Mediterranean

Military hospital ships have their function to transport the sick and wounded from overseas ports where the casualties are received on board from the ambulance trains. These military H.S. are only brought into action when the occasion demands it and are not a permanent part of the military force. Hospital ships used by the military are painted all white with a horizontal green band about 5 feet wide surrounding the ship's hull. Private hospital ships are also active, donated by various societies, such as the Red Cross, were also distinguishable painted all white with a broad red band around the ship's hull. Red Crosses appeared on all hospital ships, on their sides, fore and aft and amidships, as well as flying the Red Cross flag with their individual national flag.

The Red Cross

This is the brief story of the foundation of the great movement which, as a worldwide organisation, conducts a marvellous service to humanity.

There was no reason to doubt the impact on Henri Dunant's mind of what he had seen on the battlefields during his travels. In those days of rough surgery, without drugs or anaesthetics, the sights and the suffering must have been appalling.

Dunant concluded that it should be possible to form relief societies to train volunteers to nurse, comfort and care for the wounded in wartime. These societies could be based upon some principle internationally agreed at conferences and with a set of objectives laid down. The rules drawn up resulting from the objectives should be made binding in case of any conflict. It would really go further and assist refugees often left without aid after a war was concluded.

Henri Dunant put all his thoughts on paper and brought them togther into a book published in 1862. Copies of this were sent to crowned heads, princes, ministers of war and foreign affairs, to everyone he thought might be of importance in Europe. The book proved to be a sensation. A lawyer named Gustave Moynier read it and was impressed enough to visit Dunant.

The first question Moynier asked when they met was - what had he done to investigate his ideas and put them into motion? Dunant's answer was that he considered it was the international powers who should take the necessary action, but Moynier did not agree that one should wait for others to act, so he joined forces with Dunant, pushing him into action himself. This was the seed that was to grow into the International Red Cross.

Moynier was the Chairman of the Geneva Public Welfare Society and he approached them to appoint a committee whose task it would be to prepare a memorandum on the proposed relief societies. Besides Moynier and Dunant, who also acted as the secretary, there were three other members; General Dufour a strategist admired throughout Europe; Dr Appia, a war surgeon, and Dr Maunior, a fine surgeon. Gustav Moynier proposed a plan that they should themselves convene a conference of the states and their experts to consider the role of relief societies and their acceptance by the military authorities.

Henri Dunant went to Berlin to meet a Dutch military doctor, Dr Basting: from their meeting Dunant had a vague idea of some international principle developing into a concept of a convention agreed by countries, giving medical personnel a new status of 'neutrality'. Dunant issued a circular letter convening the conference and explaining his plan. He worked hard to get countries to send representatives by travelling extensively, particularly in France and Germany.

Moynier thought Dunant was asking for something that was impossible, but he was proved to be wrong. The conference held in 1863 was quite a success, 36 people being delegates from 14 states, including Great Britain, attended. Dunant's ideas were debated and finally ten resolutions were passed for the organisation and operation of relief societies, the Geneva Committee to act as a communicating link for international meetings and, as a separate matter from the resolutions, the vital recommendation on the neutrality of the Army Medical Services and those under their care. Once more the Committee shouldered the responsibility to act on these resolutions. The Swiss federal Council agreed to convene a diplomatic conference, but only providing the Committee would undertake all arrangements.

A convention was drafted by Moynier and Dunant on 22nd August, 1864, the delegates from 12 nations signed the 'Convention of Geneva for the amelioration of the condition of the wounded in the armies in the field'. The ratification by the signatories necessary to bring the Convention into force followed rapidly. By 1867 the great powers had ratified or acceded, except for the United States of America, who did so some years later, in 1882.

Dunant's original idea of voluntary relief societies had received enthusiastic backing at the Geneva Conference and gained a response in many countries. The first society was formed in 1863 and later many more started in Europe and across the world: the British Society was formed in 1870. The Geneva Committee remained in being for some time, continuing later under the name of the 'International Committee'.

From the beginning, the red cross on a white ground, the adopted emblem of the Geneva Conference, was used on uniforms and flags.

As for Henri Dunant, there is a sad tale to tell. His business ventures failed and in 1867 he was declared bankrupt and had to give up his membership of the Committee, retiring not long after into an obscurity from which he did not emerge until, as an old man, he was rediscovered in penury and had honours heaped upon him, including the Nobel Peace Prize.

St John Ambulance Association

The St John Ambulance Association is a branch of the Order of St John, whose primary mission was to care for the pilgrims and the sick, and still carries out this work.

The Order developed as the military Knights Hospitallers during the Crusades, being founded about the year 1092. They, along with the Knights Templar were the principle defence of the Christian Kingdoms in the Holy Land, but with the fall of Acre in 1291, they had to move to Cyprus, from where they captured Rhodes, ruling as a sovereign power for two hundred years. They were forced out by the Turks in 1522 and were given the island of Malta in 1530 by Charles V, Holy Roman Emperor.

When Napoleon captured Malta in 1798 the Knights Hospitaller ended their military role and, since then, have devoted themselves to humanitarian activities. According to the thirteenth statute of the Order, knights were expected to wear the familiar white pointed cross of the Order on their mantles.

The Priory in Clerkenwell, London, the headquarters of the Order of St John in England, was founded in 1140 on open ground outside the City of London. A Norman knight, Jordan de Briset, had given the land for the building of a Hospitaller Priory and a Benedictine nunnery. The first Priory building, of which only the Norman crypt now remains, were largely destroyed during the Peasants' Revolt of 1381. For four hundred years the English priory sent the Knights to the 'Convent' or headquarters, but in 1540, following Henry VIII's Act of Dissolution, the Order in this country was suppressed.

The Gatehouse, the southern and main entrance to the Priory of Clerkenwell, was built on the site of an earlier gateway in 1504 by Prior Thomas Docwra, whose arms are displayed with those of the Order under the vaulted archway. After the dissolution of the Priory, the Gatehouse fulfilled various functions. It housed the offices of the Master of the Revels during the reign of Elizabeth I and, in the 18th century, the printing works and offices of Edmund Cave, publisher of the 'Gentleman's Magazine'.

In 1874 the Gate came into the possession of the revived

Order of St John in England, the Most Venerable Order of the Hospital of St John of Jerusalem, established in England in 1831 to uphold the Hospitaller tradition of the mediaeval Order.

From St John's Gate in 1877 was launched the St John Ambulance Association by Sir John Furley and others whose objects were to train the general public and industry in first aid, nursing, child care and hygiene, as well as to provide a conveyance service to hospitals for the sick and the infirm both at home and overseas.

From this developed the St John Ambulance Brigade in 1887 at the request of many of the public who had obtained first aid certificates of the St John Ambulance Association, wishing to form a body of uniformed volunteers which would be recognised and be ready at any time to provide assistance in case of accidents and sudden illness. All the current members of the Brigade hold a First Aid Certificate and, additionally, the nurses hold a Nursing Certificate.

The Order's second charitable foundation is the St John Ophthalmic Hospital in Jerusalem. Founded in 1882, rebuilt in 1960, and designed to serve as a Consulting Ophthalmic Hospital for the Middle East it treats large numbers of patients, conducting extensive research into trachoma.

Queen Victoria's granting of a Royal Charter in 1888 made the Order a British Royal Order of Chivalry, with the sovereign as its head.

The St John Ambulance Brigade, to maintain its efficiency, has close contacts with organisations and committees like the Royal College of Nursing, the Queen's Nursing Institute, the National Council of Councils of Social Service, the Central Council for Health Education, the Royal Society for the Prevention of Accidents, the British Red Cross Society, the Women's Royal Voluntary Service, the Girl Guides' Association and other youth organisations.

Close contact is maintained with various Government departments for consultation and advice, such as the Department of Health & Social Security, Manpower Services Commission, Department of Education, Ministry of Defence, Home Office and Ministry of Aviation. More than half a million cases of first aid are treated each year by the members as part of the public duty by volunteers, in cinemas and theatres, at ceremonial parades and sporting events and any places where their services may be needed. These duties are carried out by 39,000 adult members in the United Kingdom and a total of 150,000 throughout the world. In the field of Auxiliary Nursing, part time voluntary service running into hundreds of thousands of hours annually is given to hospitals and help is also given to District Nurses. Since 1958 the Association has collaborated with the St Andrew's Ambulance Association in Scotland and the British Red Cross Society in publishing manuals on first aid and nursing, which has ensured that unform methods are adopted.

BIBLIOGRAPHY

A manual of ambulance transport. T Longmore. 1893.
Hospital ships and ambulance trains. John Plumridge. 1975.
The birth and early days of our ambulance trains in France. Col. G
A Moore, CMG, DSO, MD. 1914.